Sex without taboos

How to live a full and satisfying sex life

Veronica Fuoco

2024 ©

To all the readers,

May this book be a source of pleasure,

discovery, and spicy conversations with your partners.

"Sex is like money: only when it's too much is it enough."

John Updike

Summary

Tired of the same old routine in the bedroom?

This book is your comprehensive guide to exploring new horizons of pleasure and sensuality. You will discover the secrets to unforgettable oral sex that will drive your partner wild, and the most effective positions to reach the G-spot and experience shared moments of ecstasy.

Have you ever wondered what Tantra is and how it can lead to prolonged orgasmic experiences?

You will find all the answers in these pages, along with practical tips for improving relationship duration, overcoming premature ejaculation, and achieving multiple orgasms.

We will also address more delicate topics such as anal sex, fisting, and rope play (shibari), providing accurate information and advice on practicing them safely and consensually.

The book also explores the psychological aspects of sexuality, helping you overcome guilt associated with specific fantasies, manage the desire to have sex in public places, and talk openly with your partner about topics like cuckolding.

No matter your age or sexual orientation, this book offers you a complete and taboo-free view of sexuality, helping you live a fulfilling intimate life and build healthy and satisfying relationships.

What are the health benefits of sex?

Sex has numerous benefits for both mental and physical health, supported by a wide range of scientific studies. Here is a detailed analysis of the main benefits:

Physical health benefits

1. **Improvement of cardiovascular function:**

   Sex is a physical activity that can help improve heart health. Studies have shown that sex can reduce the risk of heart disease, improve blood circulation, and lower blood pressure.

2. **Strengthening of the immune system:**

   People who have regular sex tend to have higher levels of immunoglobulin A (IgA), an antibody that plays a crucial role in the immune system, helping fight infections.

3. **Improvement of sleep quality:**

   Orgasm releases hormones such as oxytocin and prolactin, which promote relaxation and help improve sleep quality. This effect can contribute to better cellular repair and increased energy during the day.

4. **Reduction of pain:**

During sex, especially during orgasm, the body releases endorphins, which are natural painkillers. This can help reduce various types of pain, including headaches and joint pain.

5. **Benefits for the reproductive system:**

For women, regular sex can improve pelvic floor health, reducing the risk of urinary incontinence. For men, it can reduce the risk of prostate cancer through regular ejaculation.

Does sex benefit mental health?

Yes, sex can also benefit mental health. Here are some of the ways sexual activity can positively influence mental well-being:

1. **Hormone release**

Oxytocin: Known as the love hormone, oxytocin is released during physical contact and sex, increasing the sense of bonding and intimacy with the partner.

Endorphins: These wellness hormones reduce pain and improve mood, contributing to a sense of euphoria and well-being.

Dopamine: Sex stimulates the release of dopamine, a neurotransmitter linked to pleasure and reward, enhancing the sense of gratification.

2. **Stress reduction**

Sex can reduce cortisol levels, the stress hormone, and increase, as mentioned, the production of serotonin and dopamine, neurotransmitters associated with feelings of well-being and pleasure. Physical contact and orgasms can relieve tension and anxiety, improving daily stress management.

3.   **Increase in self-esteem and confidence**

The sense of connection with the partner can increase self-confidence and personal satisfaction.

4.   **Cognitive benefits**

Sexual activity stimulates the brain, enhancing memory and cognitive function

Studies suggest that regular sexual activity may be correlated with a lower risk of dementia and cognitive decline.

What are the most common myths about sex that need to be debunked?

Here are some of the most common and widespread myths about sex that are important to debunk:

1. **Size matters most:** In reality, sexual satisfaction depends on many factors beyond the size of the genitals, such as technique, communication, and couple chemistry.

2. **Vaginal orgasm is the only true orgasm for women:** Orgasms can also be achieved through clitoral stimulation, the G-spot, or other erogenous zones.

3. **Sex life ends with age:** With proper communication and an open mind, fulfilling intimacy can be experienced at any age.

4. **Masturbation is wrong or harmful:** It is actually a healthy and natural way to explore your body and pleasure.

5. **Gay/Lesbian people are perversive or unsatisfied:** Sexual orientation does not affect the ability to have healthy and fulfilling relationships.

6. **Sex during menstruation is dirty or dangerous:** With proper hygiene precautions, it poses no risks.

7.   **Foreplay is not that important:** It is crucial for arousal, desire, and natural lubrication.

Debunking these myths helps foster a more open, aware, and healthy attitude towards sexuality in all its forms and manifestations.

What are the best ways to stimulate the clitoris?

Stimulating the clitoris is a fundamental part of sexual pleasure for many women, as it is an extremely sensitive organ with many nerve endings. Here are some common and effective techniques for clitoral stimulation:

Manual stimulation: Using fingers to stroke, rub, or massage the clitoris. Varying pressure, rhythm, and type of movement can help discover what works best. Some women prefer circular motions, while others find up-and-down or side-to-side movements more pleasurable. Using lubricant can increase comfort and pleasure.

Oral stimulation: The tongue can provide gentle but precise stimulation. Using the tip of the tongue for light and quick movements or the entire tongue for slower and more pressure can create an intense and satisfying experience.

Sex toys: Vibrators are excellent tools for clitoral stimulation, providing consistent vibrations. There are various types of vibrators designed specifically for the clitoris, such as bullet vibrators and wand vibrators. Air stimulation toys like clitoral suckers can offer unique and intense sensations.

Sex positions: Some sexual positions are particularly effective for clitoral stimulation. For example, in the missionary position, if the penetrating partner tilts their pelvis slightly, they can stimulate the clitoris with the pubic bone. The cowgirl position allows the woman to control clitoral stimulation during penetration.

Masturbation: Exploring different techniques and rhythms to discover what brings the most pleasure.

Taking time to explore without rushing, using hands, sex toys, or a combination of both.

Water stimulation: Directing the shower stream towards the clitoris can provide pleasant and consistent stimulation. Some women find this method very relaxing and intensely pleasurable.

Breathing and muscle tension: Using breathing and muscle tension to intensify pleasure.

Contracting pelvic floor muscles during stimulation can increase sensations. Practicing Kegel exercises can help strengthen these muscles and improve sensitivity and control.

Each woman is different, and what works for one person may not work for another. The key is to explore various techniques and communicate with your partner about what you like. Emphasizing the importance of communication between partners is essential for true sexual harmony.

Stimulating the clitoris can be a journey of continuous discovery, and experimentation can lead to greater awareness and sexual pleasure. Take your time and enjoy the process of exploring your body and sensations.

Do the dimensions of the clitoris vary?

Yes, the dimensions of the clitoris can vary significantly from person to person. This variability is entirely normal and depends on several genetic and physiological factors. Here are some key aspects regarding the size and structure of the clitoris:

Anatomy and structure of the clitoris

The clitoris is a highly sensitive organ, composed of several parts, including:

1. **Glans:** The visible part of the clitoris, located above the urethral opening.

2. **Corpora cavernosa:** Internal structures that extend into the body.

3. **Crura:** Branches of the clitoris that extend along the pubic bone.

4. **Vestibular bulbs:** Elongated structures situated on either side of the vaginal opening.

Size variations

1.   **Glans:** The size of the clitoral glans can vary from a few millimeters to over a centimeter in length. On average, the length of the glans is about 5-10 mm, but it can be larger or smaller.

2.   **Total Length:** The entire clitoris, including the corpora cavernosa and crura, can have a total length of approximately 7-12 cm, although most of it is internal and not visible.

Factors influencing size

1.   **Genetics:** Genetics play a significant role in the size of the clitoris. Genetic variations influence the growth and development of this organ.

2.   **Hormones:** Hormonal levels, particularly androgens like testosterone, can affect the size of the clitoris. Certain medical conditions, such as congenital adrenal hyperplasia, can lead to an increase in clitoral size.

3.   **Age and Life Stages:** The size of the clitoris can vary during different stages of a woman's life, including puberty and menopause.

Importance of variability

The variability in clitoral size is perfectly normal and does not affect sexual function or pleasure. Every clitoris, regardless of its size, is highly innervated and sensitive, making it a crucial area for sexual pleasure.

Medical considerations

If a person notices sudden changes in the size of the clitoris or has concerns about their anatomy, it is always advisable to consult a doctor or gynecologist. In some cases, variations in clitoral size may be associated with medical conditions that require attention.

Does the G-spot really exist?

The G-spot, also known as the Gräfenberg spot, exists but is not exactly a specific "spot" as often described. Rather, it is a sensitive area located on the front wall of the vagina, behind the pubic bone, and around the urethra. This area is part of the clitoral-urethral-vaginal (CUV) complex, which includes the clitoris, urethra, and the front wall of the vagina.

When stimulated, this area can lead to intense sexual pleasure for some women. However, the sensitivity and response to G-spot stimulation vary greatly among women. Some may find this area particularly erotic, while others may not experience any specific pleasure from its stimulation.

The key is to explore and communicate with your partner to understand what works best for each person, recognizing that every body is unique and responds differently to sexual stimulation.

What are the best sexual positions to stimulate the G-spot?

There are several sexual positions that can help stimulate the G-spot in the female partner:

1.   **Reverse Cowgirl Position:** The woman sits astride the man, facing his feet. This angle allows for penetration that targets the front vaginal wall where the G-spot is located.

2.   **Spoon Position:** Both partners lie on their sides, with the woman in front. The man can penetrate from behind and use a hand to massage the G-spot internally.

3.   **Missionary Position with Raised Legs:** The man is on top in the classic missionary position, while the woman raises and bends her legs to change the angle of penetration towards the G-spot.

4.   **Face-to-Face Sitting:** The woman sits astride the man facing him and controls the depth and angle of movement to maximize G-spot stimulation.

5.   **Edge of the Bed Position:** Similar to missionary but with the woman lying on the edge of the bed or couch and the man standing in front of her. This particular angle favors contact with the G-spot.

Using vibrators or specific G-spot stimulators can also be an option.

Is it possible to have multiple orgasms and how?

Yes, having multiple orgasms is possible for some individuals, both men and women, although women seem to have a greater physiological capacity in this regard. Here are some tips that can help achieve multiple orgasms:

For Women:

After the first orgasm, continue gentle stimulation while maintaining a constant rhythm without interruptions.

Vary the types of stimulation such as penetration, clitoral stimulation, vaginal, and G-spot stimulation.

Maintain a deep state of arousal through breathing, relaxation, and erotic fantasies.

Some suggest "riding" the contractions of the previous orgasm to facilitate reaching the next one.

For Men:

Slow down arousal before orgasm to delay it and maintain the erection after the first orgasm.

Change rhythm, position, or type of stimulation after the first orgasm to reduce sensitivity.

Incorporate massage and stimulation of the perineal and prostate areas.

Practice pelvic muscle exercises for greater control.

In general, the key seems to be maintaining a state of deep physical and mental arousal before, during, and after the first orgasm. Remember that not everyone experiences multiple orgasms easily.

Why do some women not reach orgasm?

There are many reasons why some women do not reach orgasm, and these can vary greatly from person to person. One of the most common causes is the lack of knowledge about one's own body and erogenous zones. Masturbation and personal exploration can help discover what feels good and what works to achieve sexual pleasure.

A significant factor is the psychological component. Stress, anxiety, depression, and relationship problems can interfere with the ability to relax and enjoy the moment. The pressure to reach orgasm can also have the opposite effect, creating a cycle of anxiety that makes it more difficult to reach climax.

The quality of communication with a partner plays a crucial role. If women do not feel comfortable talking openly about their sexual needs and preferences, they may struggle to guide their partner towards what satisfies them. Lack of adequate stimulation, such as insufficient attention to the clitoris, which is a primary source of pleasure for many women, can be an obstacle.

Physical and medical factors can also influence. Issues such as insufficient lubrication, infections, chronic medical conditions, or side effects of certain medications can negatively affect the ability to reach orgasm.

Additionally, past negative sexual experiences or trauma can have a lasting impact on sexual response.

Finally, misinformation or unrealistic expectations about sexuality, often fueled by media and pornography, can lead to frustration and dissatisfaction. It's important to have a realistic and healthy view of sex, understanding that every body is different and that the path to orgasm can vary greatly.

In many cases, the solution may include a combination of sexual education, improved communication with the partner, relaxation techniques, and if necessary, sexual counseling or therapy to address deeper issues. Recognizing and addressing these factors can help women improve their sexual lives and reach orgasm more frequently and satisfyingly.

Is it possible to fake an orgasm without the partner noticing?

It is possible to fake an orgasm quite convincingly, but it is not advisable in a healthy relationship based on trust and open communication.

Here are some factors to consider:

The physical signs of a real orgasm, such as rhythmic contractions, flushing, lubrication, and changes in breathing, are difficult to perfectly imitate.

An attentive and experienced partner may notice small inconsistencies in behavior and unauthentic sounds.

Constant faking can create frustration, insecurity, and long-term intimacy problems for both partners.

Honest communication about desires, necessary foreplay, and the right stimulation is preferable to resorting to faking.

If there are problems reaching orgasm, it is better to talk about it openly without embarrassment to find solutions together.

A fulfilling sexual relationship depends on mutual understanding, not on faking. With honesty and a constructive attitude, new paths to pleasure for both can be explored, improving the couple's intimacy.

How can one overcome the problem of premature ejaculation?

Here are some tips that can help overcome the problem of premature ejaculation:

Squeeze technique exercises: During masturbation, stop stimulation just before ejaculation, wait for the sensation to diminish, and then resume. This helps control the ejaculatory reflex.

Strengthening pelvic floor muscles:

Kegel Exercises: These exercises involve contracting and relaxing the muscles that control urine flow. To find the right muscles, try stopping the flow while urinating and feel the muscles contract - these are the pelvic floor muscles. Contract these muscles, hold the contraction for 5 seconds, and relax for 5 seconds. Repeat 10-20 times several times a day. This exercise is also mentioned later in the book and is very useful for women as well.

Bridge Exercise: Lie on your back, bend your knees, and plant your feet firmly on the ground. Lift your hips by raising the pelvis upward, forming a straight line from your knees to your shoulders. Hold for a few seconds and slowly relax.

Squats: With your feet about shoulder-width apart, bend your knees, pushing your hips back as if to sit down. Keep your back straight and do not bend your knees beyond your feet. Do 10-15 repetitions.

Leg Raises: While lying on your back, lift one leg at a time, extending it upward while keeping the thigh still. Hold for a few seconds and then lower with control. Do 10-15 repetitions per leg.

It is important to perform these exercises regularly to achieve results and improve the strength and tone of the pelvic floor. In case of problems or pain, consult a physiotherapist.

Deep breathing techniques: Inhaling slowly and deeply during arousal can help delay ejaculation.

Using thick/delay condoms: These can slightly decrease penile sensitivity, delaying orgasm.

Behavioral changes: Varying the rhythm and sexual positions can help improve duration. Positions that reduce direct stimulation, such as the spoon position (both partners lie on their sides, facing the same direction. Usually, the partner behind wraps their body around the one in front, like two spoons stacked. This position allows for rear penetration, which can be vaginal or anal. It promotes great physical contact and a sense of protection and affection. Pillows can be used for added comfort, placed between the legs or under the head. The position can be easily modified to find the most comfortable angle for both partners. The spoon position is appreciated for its simplicity and intimacy, making it a popular choice for both cuddling and sexual intimacy). Changing positions during intercourse not only offers new sensations but can also help reduce the intensity of stimulation, prolonging the act.

Having sex twice in a short time: After the first intercourse, it is easier to control ejaculation the second time.

Behavioral therapy: An experienced therapist can teach targeted cognitive-behavioral techniques.

Medications: In severe cases, antidepressants or topical anesthetics may be prescribed, but only under strict medical supervision.

Lifestyle changes: Reducing stress, improving communication with the partner, and maintaining a healthy sexual life can have positive effects.

Avoiding alcohol and drugs: These substances can negatively affect sexual performance and worsen the problem.

Remember that it is always advisable to consult a healthcare professional for a personalized evaluation and to explore the most suitable options for your case.

What are the secrets to a simultaneous orgasm with a partner?

Achieving a simultaneous orgasm with a partner is one of the most fulfilling experiences in a couple's sexual life. Although it may require practice and synchronization, it is not an unattainable goal. The key lies in open communication, mutual understanding of sexual rhythms, and the ability to tune in to each other's desires and needs.

First and foremost, it is essential to openly talk with your partner about your expectations and desires. Discussing fantasies, pleasure points, and preferences can help create an environment of intimacy and mutual understanding. Knowing the times and ways in which each partner reaches orgasm is fundamental. Some may prefer slow and gradual stimulation, while others may find a faster pace more exciting.

Another crucial aspect is the prelude to the actual sexual act. Foreplay plays an important role in synchronizing both partners' arousal levels. Take the time to explore each other's bodies using kisses, caresses, and other forms of stimulation. This not only increases arousal but also helps create a deeper emotional bond, which can facilitate achieving a simultaneous orgasm.

During intercourse, it is useful to pay attention to the partner's body signals. Communicating through moans, movements, and words can help understand when the other is close to climax. Adjusting the rhythm and intensity of penetration or stimulation can help keep both partners on the same level of arousal. If one partner approaches orgasm faster, they can slow down slightly to allow the other to catch up.

Sexual positions can also make a difference. Some positions favor more intense and simultaneous contact of erogenous zones. For example, the missionary position allows for good visual and physical contact, while the spoon position (explained earlier) can facilitate simultaneous stimulation of the clitoris and penis.

The use of sex toys can be a great ally. Vibrators and other devices can provide additional stimulation, helping to synchronize the timing of orgasms. Integrating them into foreplay or during intercourse can intensify the experience and increase the chances of a simultaneous climax.

Finally, it is important not to be overwhelmed by the pressure of achieving a simultaneous orgasm. The primary goal should be mutual pleasure and emotional connection. Achieving a simultaneous orgasm is wonderful, but it should not become an obsession or source of stress. With practice, patience, and communication, you can discover new dimensions of pleasure together and ultimately experience moments of shared ecstasy.

The secret to a simultaneous orgasm with your partner lies in mutual understanding and the ability to tune into each other's desires. With time and exploration, you can achieve this fulfilling experience and further strengthen your bond.

Does penis size matter?

The question of penis size and its importance is a topic that generates a lot of interest and debate. It's important to approach this subject in a balanced and informed manner, considering both physical and psychological and relational aspects.

Physical aspects:

From a physical standpoint, the size of the penis has a variable impact on sexual satisfaction. Most of the nerve endings sensitive to pleasure are located in the first few centimeters inside the vagina, and many sexual positions can be adapted to maximize pleasure regardless of penis length. Additionally, the width or girth of the penis may be more relevant for some people compared to length, as it can influence the sensation of fullness during penetration.

Psychological aspects:

The importance attributed to penis size is often influenced by psychological and cultural factors. Society and the media tend to emphasize certain ideals of masculinity that can make men feel insecure about their size. These insecurities can negatively affect self-esteem and sexual confidence, regardless of the actual ability to satisfy a partner.

It's important to recognize that sexual confidence and competence do not solely depend on penis size. Communication, consideration for the partner, and the ability to explore and understand each other's desires and preferences play a fundamental role in sexual satisfaction.

Relational aspects:

In a relationship, sexual satisfaction is the result of a combination of factors, including emotional intimacy, communication, and the ability to respond to the partner's needs. Many people report that emotional connection and sexual compatibility are much more important than penis size.

Exploring different sexual positions, using sex toys, and other forms of stimulation can enrich a couple's sex life regardless of penis size.

Research and studies:

Scientific research shows that for most people, penis size is not the main factor for sexual satisfaction. Studies have demonstrated that the vast majority of heterosexual women are satisfied with their partner's penis size and that other aspects of the relationship and sexual behavior are much more influential on overall satisfaction.

While penis size may play a role in individual preferences, it is not the determining factor for sexual satisfaction or a fulfilling sexual relationship. Emotional intimacy, understanding each other's desires, and the ability to adapt and respond to the partner's needs are all fundamental elements for a satisfying sex life. It is important to focus on these aspects rather than physical dimensions to build a fulfilling and lasting sexual and relational connection.

What are the ideal penis dimensions?

The question of ideal penis dimensions is surrounded by many myths and misunderstandings. As already explained in the previous answer, penis size is much less important than often believed. Instead, many other elements play a more significant role.

First, sexual compatibility and emotional intimacy are crucial for a satisfying sexual experience. Mutual respect and attention to the partner's desires and needs are fundamental. Couples who communicate well and are emotionally close tend to have a more fulfilling sex life, regardless of penis size.

Second, sexual technique and skill are much more important than size. The ability to stimulate the partner in different ways, to be attentive, and to respond to their reactions significantly contributes to sexual satisfaction. Knowledge of the partner's body and erogenous zones can have a much greater impact than the length or girth of the penis.

Moreover, many women find that penis girth is more relevant than length for internal stimulation. However, most female sexual pleasure derives from clitoral stimulation, which can be achieved in many different ways, not necessarily related to penetration.

Insecurities related to penis size often stem from unrealistic standards promoted by the media and pornography. These representations do not reflect the reality of most people and can create unrealistic expectations. It's important to remember that every body is different and that there is a wide range of normality when it comes to penis size.

Finally, the average size of an erect penis is generally between 12 and 16 centimeters, with significant variations still falling within the norm. Most men fall within this range and have no reason to worry excessively about their size.

In conclusion, the truth about ideal penis size is that there is no universal ideal measurement. Sexual satisfaction depends much more on emotional compatibility, communication, technique, and mutual attention rather than physical dimensions. Accepting and appreciating one's body and that of the partner is fundamental for a healthy and fulfilling sex life.

Does penis size change with age?

Yes, the size of the penis can change with age due to various physiological and hormonal factors. These changes can affect both the length and girth of the penis. Here is a detailed overview of how and why the size of the penis may vary throughout life:

Changes during life

Adolescence

Pubertal Growth: During puberty, the penis undergoes significant growth due to increased testosterone levels. This growth phase can last several years, generally from ages 10 to 18.

Adulthood

Stability: Once sexual maturity is reached, around ages 18-21, the size of the penis tends to stabilize. During young and middle adulthood, no significant changes in penis size usually occur.

Aging

Reduction in Size: As men age, some may notice a slight reduction in penis size, both when flaccid and erect. This change is gradual and can be influenced by various factors:

Decrease in Testosterone: Testosterone levels tend to decline with age, which can affect muscle mass and bone density, including penile tissues.

Loss of Tissue Elasticity: The elastic tissues of the penis may lose elasticity and tone, leading to a reduction in length and girth.

Plaque Accumulation: Plaque can accumulate in the blood vessels of the penis (a condition known as Peyronie's disease), causing curvature and potentially reducing length.

Increase in Fat Tissue: An increase in abdominal fat can make the penis appear smaller due to partial coverage by pubic fat.

Factors influencing penis size

Lifestyle and general health

Body Weight: Being overweight can affect the perceived size of the penis. Reducing body fat can make the penis appear larger.

Physical Activity: Maintaining good physical fitness and healthy blood circulation is important for penile health.

Smoking and Alcohol: Smoking and excessive alcohol use can negatively affect blood circulation and erectile function.

Medical Issues

Erectile dysfunction: Difficulty maintaining an erection can make the penis appear smaller.

Cardiovascular Diseases: Conditions that affect blood circulation can influence the ability to achieve and maintain an erection.

Psychological considerations

The perception of penis size can be influenced by psychological and cultural factors. Performance anxiety and concerns about size can affect personal perception and sexual satisfaction.

Can women ejaculate?

Yes, women can ejaculate. This phenomenon is known as "female ejaculation" and is often confused with "squirting." Here is a detailed explanation:

Female Ejaculation

What it is:

Female ejaculation is the release of fluid from the Skene's glands, located around the urethra. These glands are sometimes called the "female prostate" because they produce a fluid similar to male prostatic fluid.

Quantity and appearance:

The amount of fluid can vary from a few drops to a small visible amount. The fluid is generally clear or milky and has a different consistency from urine.

Chemical composition:

The fluid from female ejaculation contains components similar to male prostatic fluid, such as prostatespecific antigen (PSA) and prostatic acid phosphatase (PAP).

Squirting

What it is:

Squirting is the expulsion of a larger amount of fluid that occurs during orgasm or intense sexual arousal. The fluid comes mainly from the bladder and is mostly diluted urine.

Quantity and appearance:

The amount of fluid can be quite large, similar to that of urination. The fluid is usually clear and may have a urine-like odor, though it is more diluted.

Differences between female ejaculation and squirting

Origin: Female ejaculation comes from the Skene's glands, while the fluid from squirting comes from the bladder.

Composition: The fluid from female ejaculation contains PSA and PAP, while the fluid from squirting is mostly diluted urine.

Considerations

Normalcy and variations:

Not all women experience female ejaculation or squirting, and the presence or absence of these phenomena does not indicate anything abnormal or problematic. Every woman is different and responds uniquely to sexual stimulation.

Experience and stimulation:

Stimulation of the G-spot or intense arousal can increase the likelihood of experiencing female ejaculation or squirting. However, there are no universal techniques that work for everyone.

Research and awareness:

Research on female ejaculation and squirting is ongoing, and there is growing awareness and acceptance of these phenomena in society.

How important is oral sex in a relationship?

Oral sex can play a significant role in a relationship, but its importance varies from couple to couple. For many, oral sex is a form of intimacy and pleasure that enriches their sexual life and contributes to a sense of connection and mutual satisfaction. It can be a way to explore a partner's sexuality, increase variety, and keep the passion alive.

From a pleasure standpoint, oral sex offers different kinds of stimulation compared to penetrative sex, allowing each partner to discover new ways to reach orgasm and experience pleasure. For some individuals, oral sex can be particularly pleasurable or even necessary to achieve orgasm.

Communication is crucial when it comes to oral sex, just as it is for any other aspect of sexual life. Openly discussing preferences, desires, and boundaries can help create an environment of trust and respect, making the experience more enjoyable for both partners. It's important that both partners feel comfortable giving and receiving oral sex, and that no one feels obligated to engage in it.

In addition to physical pleasure, oral sex can strengthen the emotional bond between partners. The vulnerability and intimacy involved in this practice can contribute to greater connection and mutual understanding. However, it's important to remember that every couple is different, and what works for one couple may not be as significant for another.

What are the secrets to unforgettable oral sex?

To make oral sex an unforgettable experience, the main key is connection and communication with your partner. Each person has different preferences, so openly discussing likes and dislikes can make a big difference. Trust and comfort are fundamental for fully letting go and enjoying the experience.

Awareness of your own body and your partner's body is another crucial aspect. Take the time to explore and understand your partner's reactions. Every small response, whether it's a moan, a deeper breath, or a body movement, can provide valuable clues about what's working and what's not. This type of attention and sensitivity makes oral sex more personal and engaging.

Variety in techniques and rhythms can keep the excitement high. Alternating speeds, pressure, and movements can create complex and surprising stimulation, enhancing pleasure. Eye contact and the use of hands can also amplify the intimacy and intensity of the moment. Hands can be used to caress other parts of the body or to increase stimulation in sync with the mouth.

Additionally, don't underestimate the importance of foreplay. Creating a relaxed and sensual atmosphere with kisses, caresses, and whispered words can prepare your partner and increase anticipation.

This emotional and physical preparation makes oral sex even more fulfilling.

Integrate different stimulations such as massaging the external genitals, the perineum, and the anal area if desired. Maintain intimate hygiene for greater disinhibition for both partners.

Be creative and open to new positions and angles. Afterwards, continue with cuddles, kisses, and tenderness for a greater sense of connection. Finally, pleasure during oral sex is not only about the partner who receives it. Find pleasure in giving, enjoying the reactions and satisfaction of your partner. This mutual exchange of pleasure and attention is what makes oral sex truly memorable and unique.

Remember that every couple is different, and what works for one may not work for another. The key is to be present, attentive, and always ready to learn and adapt to your partner's needs and desires.

What does swallowing sperm involve?

Swallowing sperm does not pose health risks from a medical perspective. Sperm is mainly composed of fluids produced by male sexual glands and contains nutrients like fructose, proteins, zinc, and other molecules. Unless there are sexually transmitted infections (STIs) present, swallowing semen itself is not dangerous.

However, the act of swallowing sperm can evoke different psychological and emotional reactions from person to person, influenced by cultural, religious, personal factors, or individual tastes/disgust. Some people consider it natural and intimate, while others feel disgusted.

From a sexual safety perspective, if both partners are healthy and free of STIs, there are no specific medical contraindications. But it remains a very personal and intimate choice, to be approached with respect, without coercion, and based on mutual consent and comfort.

Aphrodisiacs are substances believed to increase sexual desire, pleasure, or performance. However, scientific evidence regarding their effectiveness is often limited or controversial. Many aphrodisiacs have a psychological rather than physiological effect, influencing desire and arousal mainly through the power of suggestion.

Here is an overview of some common aphrodisiacs and the evidence related to their effectiveness:

Chocolate: Contains phenylethylamine and serotonin, chemicals that can improve mood. However, there is no solid evidence that it increases sexual desire.

Oysters: Rich in zinc, which is important for testosterone production. However, there is no direct evidence that oysters increase sexual desire.

Honey: Contains boron, which can help regulate hormone levels. However, evidence of its effectiveness as an aphrodisiac is anecdotal.

Ginseng: Some studies suggest that ginseng may improve sexual function, but the results are mixed and not definitive.

Maca: A Peruvian root that some studies have associated with increased sexual desire, although further research is needed.

Aphrodisiacs with Some Scientific Evidence

1. Tribulus Terrestris:

- Some studies suggest it may increase testosterone levels and improve libido, but the evidence is still inconclusive.

2. Ginkgo Biloba:

- May improve blood circulation, including to the genitals, potentially enhancing sexual function.

3. Yohimbine:

- Derived from the bark of the Yohimbe tree, some studies have shown an improvement in male sexual dysfunctions. However, it can have significant side effects such as anxiety and high blood pressure.

Common Natural Aphrodisiacs

1. **Spices** (ginger, cinnamon, nutmeg):

- Can improve circulation and have stimulating properties. The aphrodisiac effect is mostly anecdotal.

2. **Avocado**:

- Rich in vitamin E, potassium, and vitamin B6, which are important for sexual health.

3. **Pomegranate**:

- Contains antioxidants that can improve blood flow and vascular health.

Final considerations

Placebo and Suggestion: Many aphrodisiacs work primarily through the placebo effect and the power of suggestion. Believing that a substance can increase sexual desire can actually enhance arousal and pleasure.

Safety: Before trying any aphrodisiac, especially those less known or with potential side effects, it's important to consult a doctor.

Lifestyle: A balanced diet, regular exercise, stress reduction, and good communication with your partner are fundamental for a healthy sex life.

**How can sex be made more exciting after years of relationship?**

Making sex more exciting after years of relationship requires creativity, communication, and a willingness to explore new experiences together. One of the first things to do is to talk openly with your partner about your fantasies and desires. Often, after years of being together, people assume they know everything about each other, but desires and preferences can evolve. Honest communication can reveal new aspects of sexuality that have not yet been explored.

Another strategy is to experiment with new sexual activities. Trying new positions, role-playing, using sex toys, or exploring different environments can add a sense of novelty and adventure. Even simple changes, like making love in a different room of the house or spending more time on foreplay, can make a big difference.

Maintaining spontaneity is crucial. Although daily life is full of commitments, finding moments for intimacy without overly planning them can make sex more exciting. Letting yourself go in the moment, perhaps surprising your partner with affectionate and spontaneous gestures, can rekindle passion.

Emotional involvement is equally important. Strengthening the emotional bond through shared activities that are not necessarily sexual, such as romantic walks, candlelit dinners, or trips together, can improve the sexual connection. Feeling emotionally close and appreciated facilitates deeper and more satisfying intimacy.

Finally, do not underestimate the power of self-care. Maintaining a healthy lifestyle, feeling good about your body, and cultivating self-esteem can positively impact your sex life. When you feel comfortable with yourself, it is easier to let go and enjoy intimacy with your partner.

What are the best role-playing games to try in the bedroom?

Role-playing games in the bedroom can add an exciting and fun dimension to a couple's sex life. They allow partners to explore fantasies, roles, and power dynamics in a safe and consensual environment. Here are some of the best role-playing games to try, each with suggestions to make them enjoyable and stimulating.

1. **Student and Teacher:** This classic role-playing game explores the power dynamics between an authority figure (the teacher) and a subordinate (the student). The partner playing the teacher can give "lessons" or assign "homework" to the student, who may have to "earn" good grades through various activities.

    To make the experience more authentic, you can dress according to the roles, using appropriate clothing like a pleated skirt and blouse for the student and a formal outfit for the teacher. Communication is essential to set limits and ensure both partners are comfortable.

2. **Police Officer and Criminal:** In this scenario, one partner plays the police officer who must arrest or interrogate the criminal. This role-playing game can include the use of toy

handcuffs, uniforms, and interrogations. The dynamics of capture and control can be very exciting and allow partners to explore themes of submission and dominance.

Establishing a safe word is particularly important in this type of game to ensure everything happens with mutual respect and comfort.

3.   **Doctor and Patient:** The doctor and patient role-playing game allows you to explore themes of care and trust. The partner playing the doctor can perform a "check-up," which can include massages, "exams," and various treatments.

This scenario is perfect for those who enjoy physical contact and the feeling of being cared for or caring for their partner. Tools like a toy stethoscope, thermometer, and lab coat can make the game more realistic and engaging.

4.   **Strangers in a Bar:** This role-playing game begins with both partners pretending not to know each other and meeting for the first time in a bar or another public place. You can start at home, perhaps sharing a drink together and exchanging flirtatious banter as strangers. This game allows you to reignite the spark of the beginning of a relationship and can lead to very passionate interactions.

The fun lies in creating new identities and flirting as if you were perfect strangers. This roleplaying game is particularly useful for breaking the routine and rediscovering the excitement of seduction.

5.   **Master and Submissive:** The Master and Submissive role-playing game is part of the BDSM world and is based on dominance and submission dynamics. The dominant partner (Master) gives orders and controls the situation, while the submissive partner obeys. This game requires strong communication and a high level of mutual trust.

Before starting, it is important to discuss each other's limits and fantasies, establishing safe words to ensure both partners can stop the game at any time. Accessories like whips, ropes, and masks can add authenticity to the role.

6.   **Fantasy Characters:** Playing fantasy characters like vampires, aliens, or superheroes can be extremely fun and stimulating. These role-playing games allow you to explore imaginary worlds and play with extraordinary powers and abilities.

Costumes, makeup, and settings can help you get into character and make the experience more engaging. This type of role-playing game is perfect for those with a vivid imagination and a love for fantasy stories.

Role-playing games in the bedroom offer endless possibilities for exploring new dynamics and spicing up your sex life. With creativity and respect, role-playing games can lead to unforgettable experiences and strengthen the bond between partners.

How long should a sexual encounter last to be satisfying?

The ideal duration of a sexual encounter varies from couple to couple and depends on many factors, including personal preferences, the type of stimulation, and the emotional interaction between partners. However, a study by the Society for Sex Therapy and Research in Washington found that the most pleasing duration for couples to make love is between 7-13 minutes. Beyond 13 minutes, distractions and fatigue can decrease desire, while within seven minutes, it is likely that at least one of the partners will remain unsatisfied.

It is important to note that sexual satisfaction does not depend solely on the duration of penetrative sex. Other factors such as foreplay, the quality of stimulation, and emotional intimacy play a crucial role in achieving sexual pleasure. Therefore, instead of focusing exclusively on duration, it is essential to pay attention to the overall quality of the sexual experience, ensuring that both partners feel comfortable and satisfied.

What is bondage and how can it be introduced into a sexual relationship?

Bondage is a sexual practice that involves the use of ropes, straps, handcuffs, or other tools to immobilize or tie up the partner, creating a dynamic of power and control. Often associated with BDSM (Bondage, Discipline, Dominance, Submission, Sadism, Masochism), bondage can be a form of erotic expression and a way to explore trust and connection between partners. Here's how to introduce bondage into a sexual relationship safely and consensually.

Understanding Bondage

First of all, it's important to understand what bondage entails. It's not just about physically tying someone up but creating a shared experience that can be both physical and mental. Bondage can range from simple and decorative ties to more complex and restrictive scenarios, always with the aim of exploring new dynamics of pleasure and connection.

Communicating with your partner

The first step to introducing bondage into your relationship is communication. Talk to your partner about your fantasies and curiosities regarding bondage. Listen to their thoughts and feelings about it as well. It's essential that both of you are open and honest during this conversation. Discuss what excites you, what you feel comfortable with, and the limits that both of you want to set.

Establishing limits and consent

Once both of you have expressed interest, it's important to establish clear limits and obtain consent. Consent must be enthusiastic and continuous. This means that both parties should feel free to express their desires and say "no" at any time. Establish "safe words" that can be used to immediately stop the activity if either of you feels uncomfortable.

Educating yourself on safety techniques

Bondage, like all BDSM practices, requires knowledge of safety techniques. Educate yourselves on the basics of bondage, such as avoiding tying too tightly to prevent injuries or circulation problems. You can find resources online, in books, or through workshops dedicated to these techniques. Safety must always be the priority.

Starting with basic equipment

When you're ready to start, begin with simple and easy-to-use equipment. Padded handcuffs, silk straps, or ropes specifically designed for bondage are good options for beginners. Avoid complex tools until you have gained more experience and confidence in your abilities.

Creating the right atmosphere

Creating a relaxed and intimate atmosphere can help both of you feel more at ease. Use soft lighting, relaxing music, and ensure that everything you need is within reach. Take the time to talk and relax before starting, making sure both of you are ready and eager to explore together.

Practicing with care and respect

When you start practicing bondage, do it with care and respect. Begin with simple ties and gradually explore more advanced techniques as both of you feel comfortable. Communicate continuously during the activity to ensure both of you are enjoying the experience.

Reflecting on the experience

After the session, take some time to talk about how it went. Discuss what you liked, what could be improved, and any feelings or emotions that emerged. This helps build trust and improve future experiences.

Bondage can be an exciting and rewarding addition to your sexual life, strengthening the connection and trust between you and your partner. The key is always open communication, consent, and careful consideration of safety. With time and practice, bondage can become a natural and enjoyable part of your sexual relationship, allowing you to explore new dimensions of pleasure and intimacy.

What is and how can rope play (shibari) be introduced into your sexual life?

Rope play, also known as *shibari* or *kinbaku*, is an ancient Japanese practice that involves the art of tying the body with ropes in an artistic and erotic way. This practice can add a new and intensely intimate dimension to a couple's sexual life, as it involves not only physical stimulation but also emotional and mental connection.

To introduce *shibari* into your sexual life, the first fundamental step is open communication with your partner. Talk about your fantasies and desires, explaining why you are interested in exploring this practice. It's important that both of you agree and feel comfortable with the idea. Discussing limits and expectations is essential to ensure that the experience is safe and enjoyable for both.

Once mutual interest is established, it's helpful to educate yourselves on the subject. Reading books, watching tutorial videos, and attending workshops can provide a good knowledge base. *Shibari* requires skill and attention to safety, so it's important to learn the correct techniques and understand the associated risks. Ropes should be used in a way that does not cause pain or injury, and you need to be aware of the areas of the body that are more sensitive or at risk.

When you are ready to start, choose a quiet and comfortable environment where you can fully dedicate yourselves to this practice without interruptions. Ensure that you have everything you need at hand: suitable ropes, safety scissors for emergencies, and if necessary, a mat or pillows for the partner's comfort.

Start with simple and basic ties that are easier to execute and less risky. Maintain continuous communication throughout the process, asking your partner how they feel and if something is wrong. Trust is the foundation of shibari, and each tie should be done with care and attention.

As you gain confidence and skill, you can experiment with more complex and artistic ties. Shibari is not just a sexual practice but also a visual art; the ties can be beautiful to look at and can add an aesthetic element to your intimacy.

Finally, it is important to reflect on the experience after the session. Talk about what you liked, what could be improved, and how you felt. This helps strengthen the connection between you and your partner and improve future experiences.

Shibari can be a wonderful and deeply intimate addition to your sexual life, offering new opportunities for exploration and connection. With proper preparation, communication, and attention to safety, this practice can lead to greater mutual understanding and pleasure.

How often is it normal to desire sex?

Sexual desire varies greatly from person to person and can be influenced by a number of factors, including age, health, stress levels, relationship quality, psychological and hormonal factors, and lifestyle. There is no universal "normal" frequency for sexual desire, as what is normal varies significantly from individual to individual.

Some people may have a strong sexual desire and think about sex frequently, perhaps every day or even multiple times a day. Other people may have a less frequent sexual desire, desiring sex only once a week, a month, or even less often. Both situations can be perfectly normal if they correspond to the individual's preferences and well-being.

Sexual desire can also fluctuate over the course of life and in response to different situations. For example, desire may increase during periods of new infatuation or great intimacy and decrease during periods of stress, illness, or relationship tensions. Fluctuations are part of the normal human experience.

It is important to recognize and accept your own level of sexual desire without judgment. The key is to understand if your level of sexual desire is in harmony with your well-being and the quality of your relationship. If a person is satisfied with their frequency of desire and their sex life, it is likely that it is "normal" for them.

In a relationship, differences in levels of sexual desire between partners can be a source of conflict. It is essential to have open and honest communication about your desires and needs. Compromises and creative solutions can help balance the differences, such as finding other forms of intimacy and connection that satisfy both partners.

If a person or couple experiences a significant discrepancy in sexual desire that causes discomfort or dissatisfaction, it may be helpful to seek the help of a professional, such as a sex therapist or couples counselor. These experts can offer support and strategies for managing and harmonizing levels of sexual desire.

In summary, there is no universal "normal" frequency for sexual desire. It is normal for people to have different levels of sexual desire and for these to change over time. The most important thing is that the level of sexual desire is in harmony with your well-being and the quality of your relationship. If problems or conflicts arise, open communication and professional help can be valuable resources.

Is it possible to have an orgasm during anal sex?

Yes, it is possible to have an orgasm during anal sex. Orgasm can be achieved through various types of sexual stimulation, including anal sex. For many people, anal sex can indirectly stimulate the prostate in men (known as the "P-spot") or other erogenous zones in women. The prostate is a gland that, when stimulated, can produce intense sensations and lead to orgasm. For women, anal stimulation can also indirectly involve the G-spot and clitoris, contributing to arousal and achieving orgasm. However, it's important to note that sexual response varies from person to person. Open communication and consent are essential in any sexual activity, including anal sex. Additionally, it is crucial to use appropriate lubricants and proceed slowly to ensure comfort and safety during anal sex.

Convincing a partner to try anal sex requires open, honest, and respectful communication. Here are some suggestions for addressing the topic:

1.   **Be Open and honest:** Explain why you would like to try anal sex, sharing your fantasies and desires. Being sincere about your feelings can help your partner better understand your motivations.

2.   **Listen to your partner:** Ask your partner how they feel about anal sex and listen carefully to their concerns or

fears. It's important to respect their feelings and not downplay them.

3.   **Read Information Together:** Suggest reading information about anal sex, including techniques, benefits, and necessary precautions. Being better informed can help both of you feel more comfortable.

4.   **Discuss safety and comfort:** Explain the importance of using lubricants, proceeding slowly, and listening to your partner's body. Make sure to discuss the use of condoms to prevent infections.

5.   **Propose gradual alternatives:** Suggest starting with lighter activities like external anal stimulation or using small sex toys to gradually get used to the sensation.

6.   **Always respect your partner:** Enthusiastic consent is fundamental for any sexual activity. If your partner is not interested or not ready, respect their decision without pressure.

7.   **Be patient:** Give your partner time to consider your proposal and don't expect an immediate yes. Patience and understanding are essential for building trust and security.

8.   **Maintain a positive attitude:** Avoid making your partner feel guilty or putting too much pressure on them. Be positive and reassuring, making it clear that your common goal is mutual pleasure and satisfaction.

What are the best lubricants for anal sex?

Anal sex can be a pleasurable and safe experience, especially when using an appropriate lubricant. Lubricants reduce friction, which can help prevent discomfort and injury. Here is a guide to the best types of lubricants for anal sex:

Types of lubricants

1. **Water-based lubricants:**

___ **Pros:** Easy to clean, safe to use with all types of condoms and sex toys, non-staining.

Cons: Dry out faster than other types, may need reapplication during activity.

Recommended:

K-Y Jelly: A classic option, easily available.

Sliquid H2O: A natural lubricant, free of parabens and glycerin, ideal for sensitive skin.

2. **Silicone-Based Lubricants:**

___ **Pros:** Last longer than water-based lubricants, do not require frequent reapplication, great for anal sex.

Cons: More difficult to clean, can damage silicone sex toys.

Recommended:

Pjur Original: Very popular for its long-lasting duration and silky consistency.

Wet Platinum: Known for being extremely slippery and durable.

3. **Hybrid Lubricants:**

— **Pros:** Combine the benefits of water-based and silicone lubricants, offering good duration and ease of cleaning.

Cons: May not be compatible with all silicone sex toys.

Recommended:

Sliquid Silk: A highly appreciated hybrid lubricant for its consistency and duration. **Hybrid Personal Lubricant by Good Clean Love:** Natural and free of harsh chemicals, suitable for sensitive skin.

4. **Oil-Based Lubricants:**

Pros: Long-lasting and very slippery.

Cons: Can damage latex condoms and are difficult to clean, not ideal for people with sensitive skin.

Recommended: Usually not recommended for anal sex due to potential risks of damaging condoms and cleaning difficulties.

Helpful tips

Compatibility with Condoms: If using latex condoms, avoid oil-based lubricants as they can cause breakage.

Quantity: Use a generous amount of lubricant to ensure a comfortable and pleasurable experience. **Allergic Reactions:** Always test the lubricant on a small area of skin before using it to ensure there are no allergic reactions.

The choice of the right lubricant depends on your personal preferences and specific needs. It's important to experiment to find the lubricant that offers the most comfort and pleasure during anal sex.

How can anal sex be made more pleasurable and less painful?

To make anal sex more pleasurable and less painful, here are some suggestions:

1. **Use Plenty of Lubrication:** Use water-based or silicone-based lubricants. The anal area does not produce natural lubrication, so it is essential to use plenty.

2. **Go Slowly During Initial Penetration:** Allow the sphincter to relax gradually. Never force entry.

3. **Start with Fingers or Small Toys:** Gently dilate the area before attempting full penetration.

4. **Receiver Controls Movement and Depth:** At least initially, the receiving partner should control the movement and depth to better manage any discomfort.

5. **Try Positions like Doggie Style:** This position allows for greater control.

6. **Strengthen Pelvic Muscles:** Perform exercises to strengthen the pelvic muscles for better voluntary relaxation of the sphincter.

7. **Use Low-Dose Topical Anesthetic:** If the initial opening is too sensitive, use a low-dose topical anesthetic.

8. **Double Play (Anal and Vaginal Stimulation):** Practicing anal play simultaneously with vaginal stimulation can promote relaxation.

9. **Start Already Aroused:** Being already aroused can facilitate the process.

10. **Communicate Constantly:** Stop at the slightest discomfort and communicate openly with your partner.

Patience, adequate lubrication, and careful preparation are key to making anal sex a more pleasurable rather than painful experience.

Can anal sex cause hemorrhoids?

Anal sex is not a direct cause of hemorrhoids but can aggravate an existing condition or contribute to the development of hemorrhoids in some people. Here is a detailed overview of the relationship between anal sex and hemorrhoids:

What are hemorrhoids?

Hemorrhoids are swollen blood vessels in the rectum or anus that can cause pain, itching, bleeding, and discomfort. They can be internal (inside the rectum) or external (under the skin around the anus).

Anal Sex and hemorrhoids

If not practiced correctly, anal sex can cause trauma to the anal and rectal tissues, which could aggravate hemorrhoids or contribute to their formation. Here's how:

1.   **Tissue Trauma:** Anal penetration can cause micro-lesions or trauma to the anal tissues, increasing the possibility of inflammation and swelling of the blood vessels.

2.   **Increased Pressure:** Penetration can increase pressure in the anal veins, aggravating any pre-existing hemorrhoids.

3.   **Irritation and Inflammation:** Friction and movement during anal sex can irritate and inflame existing hemorrhoids.

Precautions to Reduce Risk

To reduce the risk of irritating or aggravating hemorrhoids during anal sex, you can take several precautions:

1.   **Lubrication:** Use plenty of water-based lubricant to reduce friction and the risk of tissue trauma.

2.   **Communication and Slowness:** Communicate openly with your partner and proceed slowly to avoid trauma.

3.   **Hygiene:** Ensure the anal area is clean to prevent infections and further irritation.

4.   **Relaxation:** Ensure the anal muscles are relaxed to reduce tension and the risk of trauma.

5.   **Stop in Case of Pain:** Stop immediately if you experience pain to avoid injury.

Is it wrong to desire sex with multiple partners at the same time?

Desiring to have sex with multiple partners at the same time is not wrong, as long as all involved parties are consenting, informed, and comfortable with the situation. The desire to experiment with new sexual dynamics is natural and can vary from person to person. Ensure that all participants are fully consenting and have clearly discussed their limits and boundaries. Enthusiastic consent is fundamental in any sexual activity.

Respecting the limits and boundaries of each participant is essential. If you are new to this type of experience, start slowly and ensure you have a clear understanding of the dynamics involved. Be aware of the emotions and reactions that might emerge during and after the experience. Jealousy, insecurity, or other emotions can manifest and must be addressed with understanding and mutual support. The key is to ensure that all participants agree and feel safe and respected.

***Is it normal to have sexual fantasies about celebrities
or unattainable people?***

Yes, it is perfectly normal to have sexual fantasies about celebrities or unattainable people. Sexual fantasies are a natural part of human sexuality and can vary widely from person to person. Here are some key points to consider:

1. **Nature of Sexual Fantasies:** Sexual fantasies are a way for people to explore their desires and imagine situations they find exciting. These fantasies can involve a wide range of scenarios, including those that may not be realistic or achievable in real life.

2. **Celebrities and Unattainable People:** Fantasizing about celebrities, famous personalities, or unattainable people is common. These fantasies often have nothing to do with real intentions to act on them but rather with the attraction and allure such figures exert.

3. **Benefits of Fantasies:** Sexual fantasies can enrich one's sex life, help discover new desires, and increase arousal. They can also be a safe way to explore situations without any risk or consequence in real life.

4. **Distinguishing Fantasy from Reality:** It is important to distinguish between fantasy and reality. Sexual fantasies are a private and internal expression of desires and

do not necessarily reflect what a person actually wants to achieve.

5.   **Communicating with Your Partner:** If you feel the desire to share your fantasies with your partner, do so in an environment of trust and respect. Open communication about fantasies can enrich the couple's intimacy, but it is important to do so in a way that makes both feel comfortable.

6.   **No Judgment:** It is crucial to remember that sexual fantasies are personal, and there should be no judgment about what one finds exciting. Everyone has their own desires and imaginations, and as long as they remain within the realm of fantasy or are explored with consent and respect, they are an integral part of human sexuality.

What is fisting, and what are the risks and precautions to take?

Fisting is a sexual practice that involves inserting a hand (or sometimes both) into the partner's vagina or rectum. This practice requires significant attention to safety, communication, and consent, as it can pose significant risks if not done correctly.

Risks of Fisting

1. **Internal Injuries:**

    Inserting the hand can cause lacerations, abrasions, or perforations of the vaginal or rectal walls.

2. **Infections:**

    Introducing bacteria or other pathogens can increase the risk of infections, including sexually transmitted infections (STIs).

3. **Pain and Discomfort:**

    If not performed correctly, fisting can cause significant pain and discomfort.

4. **Bleeding:**

Internal injuries can lead to bleeding, which can be severe.

Precautions to Take

1. **Consent and Communication:**

Ensure that all participants are fully consenting and have clearly discussed their limits and boundaries. Continuous communication during the act is essential.

2. **Lubrication:**

Use plenty of lubricant to reduce friction and facilitate insertion. Water-based or silicone-based lubricants are usually recommended.

3. **Hygiene:**

Wash hands thoroughly and trim nails to avoid scratches or lacerations. Using latex gloves can add an additional layer of protection.

4. **Relaxation:**

The receiving partner should be completely relaxed. Foreplay and stimulation can help prepare the body and reduce tension.

5. **Gradual Approach:**

Start slowly and carefully, inserting one finger at a
time and always listening to the partner's feedback.
Never force the insertion.

6.   **Listening to the Body:**

Stop immediately if the receiving partner
experiences intense pain or discomfort. Safety and well-
being must be the priority.

7.   **Education:**

Educate yourself thoroughly about the practice of
fisting by reading expert guides or attending workshops
if available.

8.   **Protection:**

Use condoms on sex toys or gloves to reduce the
risk of infections. Change gloves or clean hands when
switching from anal to vaginal stimulation (or vice
versa) to avoid crosscontamination.

Final considerations

Fisting is a practice that can be very intense and requires a high
level of trust and communication between partners. If both partners
are interested and aware of the risks and precautions, it can be a
satisfying part of their sex life. However, it is essential always to
respect the partner's limits and desires, proceeding with caution and
attention to safety.

How can one overcome the sense of guilt or shame associated with specific sexual fantasies?

Overcoming the sense of guilt or shame associated with specific sexual fantasies can be challenging, but it is possible through self-reflection, education, and support. Sexual fantasies are normal and do not necessarily reflect what a person wants to do in reality. They are a way to explore desires and curiosities in a safe and controlled environment.

1. **Accepting that having fantasies is a normal part of sexuality:** Recognize that there is nothing wrong with experiencing pleasure through fantasies.

2. **Avoiding self-judgment:** Negative judgment can fuel feelings of guilt and shame.

3. **Understanding the root causes:** Ask yourself why you feel guilt or shame. Often, these feelings are rooted in cultural norms, repressive upbringing, or lack of information.

4. **Open communication:** If appropriate and comfortable, share your fantasies with your partner. Open and honest communication can strengthen the bond and reduce the sense of guilt.

5.   **Self-compassion:** Treat yourself with kindness and understanding, as you would with a dear friend. Remember that it is normal to have sexual fantasies and desires.

6.   **Recognizing diversity:** Acknowledge that human sexuality is diverse, and sexual fantasies are part of this diversity.

Is it normal to desire being dominated or dominating during sex?

Yes, it is absolutely normal to desire being dominated or dominating during sex. These desires fall under what are known as consensual power dynamics, an integral part of many sexual relationships. Often, these dynamics are expressed through practices known as BDSM (Bondage, Discipline, Dominance, Submission, Sadism, Masochism).

Human sexuality is incredibly varied and includes a wide range of fantasies and preferences. Wanting to be dominated or to dominate is just one of many expressions of sexuality and can significantly enrich a couple's sex life, creating a deeper bond and greater intimacy.

For these dynamics to be enjoyable and safe, it is crucial that everything is based on clear and enthusiastic consent. Openly discussing your fantasies and limits with your partner is essential. This communication helps establish clear boundaries and ensures that both partners feel respected and comfortable.

When exploring domination and submission desires, safety is a priority. The use of safe words is a common practice in BDSM, allowing participants to stop the activity immediately if necessary.

Educating oneself on techniques and safety practices is equally important to ensure a positive experience.

Respect and continuous communication are the foundation of these dynamics. It is crucial to respect the partner's established limits and recognize that these can change over time. Periodically discussing preferences and boundaries helps maintain consensuality and pleasure for both.

Power dynamics can increase the emotional and physical intensity of the sexual experience, offering a unique opportunity to explore different aspects of one's identity and sexual desires. However, it is important to accept and not judge one's desires. The variety of sexual fantasies is a natural part of our sexuality. If feelings of guilt or shame arise, it may be helpful to talk to a sexual therapist to better understand and accept your desires. In summary, desiring to be dominated or to dominate during sex is normal and can enrich your sex life, provided that everything happens in a context of consent, safety, and mutual respect.

How can one address the desire to have sex in public places?

The desire to have sex in public places is a fairly common sexual fantasy that many people find exciting due to its element of risk and transgression. However, there are several important considerations to keep in mind to address this desire safely and respectfully.

First of all, it is helpful to understand why you have this fantasy. For many, public sex represents an exciting break from social norms and an escape from the daily routine. The element of risk of being discovered can increase adrenaline and, consequently, sexual arousal.

If you have this desire, it is important to talk openly with your partner. Communication is key to any sexual exploration. Explain why the idea excites you and listen to your partner's feelings about it. It is essential that both of you feel comfortable with any activities you decide to undertake.

Evaluating legal risks:

Engaging in sex in public places can have significant legal consequences. In many countries, public sex is considered an obscene act, which can lead to fines, criminal charges, or even registration as a sex offender. Therefore, it is essential to be aware of local laws and potential risks.

There are ways to satisfy the desire for transgression without incurring legal risks. You could consider having sex in semi-private places, such as a secluded garden or a room with large windows but closed curtains. Another option is to recreate the feeling of "being discovered" in a safe environment, such as a vacation home or a hotel with a private balcony.

If you decide to explore sex in public places, make sure you have a safety plan. Choose times and places where you are less likely to be discovered and always have an escape plan if the situation becomes too risky.

Discretion and awareness of your surroundings are crucial.

Respect for others:

It is important to consider respect for others. Engaging in sex in places where you could be easily discovered by non-consenting people is not only risky but also disrespectful. Avoid areas frequented by families, children, or public places where the act could offend or disturb others.

How can one explore their sexuality without compromising a monogamous relationship?

Exploring your sexuality within a monogamous relationship can be a highly enriching experience that can strengthen the bond between partners while promoting personal and mutual growth. The key to doing this without compromising the relationship is open communication, shared education, and creating a safe and respectful environment.

Start by talking openly with your partner about your sexual desires and fantasies. Finding the right moment for these conversations is crucial; it is best done in a calm and intimate setting where both of you feel comfortable. The important thing is to express yourself without judgment, showing vulnerability and honesty. This not only helps to create a deeper bond but also paves the way for mutual understanding of each other's desires and needs.

At the same time, it is essential to listen carefully to what your partner has to say. Communication should be a dialogue, not a monologue. Actively listening to your partner's concerns and desires strengthens mutual trust and demonstrates respect for each other's feelings.

Another way to explore your sexuality together is through shared education. You could read books, articles, or watch documentaries on sexuality. This not only provides new ideas but also opens discussions about what might interest both of you. Attending workshops or seminars on sexuality can be an opportunity to learn together and discover new practices in a guided and safe environment.

Experimenting with new sexual practices can be a great way to explore. For example, introducing sex toys into your intimate life can add variety and stimulation. Toys such as vibrators, dildos, or cock rings can offer new sensations and pleasures. If both of you are interested, you could also explore BDSM, which can add a new dimension to your sex life through consensual power dynamics.

Trying new sexual positions can also enliven intimacy. Variety can make the experience more exciting and help discover new ways to experience pleasure. During these explorations, it is important to create a safe and respectful environment. Discussing and agreeing on which practices are acceptable and which are not is fundamental. Respecting the limits established by both partners ensures that no one feels uncomfortable or forced to do something they do not want to.

Finally, it is essential to maintain ongoing communication. Desires and boundaries can change over time, so it is helpful to have periodic conversations to review and update your preferences and limits. Patience, understanding, and mutual respect are fundamental to maintaining a healthy monogamous relationship while exploring your sexuality together.

Exploring your sexuality does not mean compromising a monogamous relationship but rather enriching it, making it deeper and more satisfying for both partners, as long as it is managed with a respectful and consensual approach.

Is it normal to desire being watched while having sex?

Yes, it is absolutely normal to desire being watched while having sex. This desire is a common sexual fantasy and can be linked to various psychological and emotional factors. Many people find the idea of being observed during intimacy exciting, a concept that falls under consensual exhibitionism. This desire can stem from the wish to feel appreciated, the search for an adrenaline rush, or the pleasure derived from transgressing social norms.

The desire to be watched can add an element of excitement and novelty to one's sex life. Knowing that someone else is watching can increase the feeling of pleasure and intensify the experience. Additionally, for some people, the idea of performing can boost self-esteem and body confidence.

It is important to remember that, like all sexual fantasies, exhibitionism must be practiced with consent and respect for all parties involved. If you wish to explore this aspect of your sexuality, the first step is to discuss it openly with your partner. Communication is fundamental to ensuring that both of you are comfortable with the idea and that you can establish clear limits and boundaries.

There are various ways to explore the desire to be watched safely and consensually. For example, you could start with lighter activities, such as having sex with the curtains open in a private but visible area or filming an intimate video to watch together. Another possibility is to participate in swinger events or private clubs where exhibitionism is accepted and practiced in a safe and consensual environment.

It is also helpful to reflect on your motivations and feelings regarding this desire. Understanding what makes being watched exciting can help integrate this fantasy into your sex life in a way that is rewarding for you and your partner. Some people may find that the desire to be watched is related to the pleasure of feeling desired and appreciated, while for others, it may be a form of exploring their sexual identity.

However, it is crucial to remember that respect and consent are at the core of every sexual practice. Never involve non-consenting people or jeopardize others' privacy and well-being. If you decide to explore exhibitionism, always ensure that all involved parties are fully aware and agreeable.

How can you talk to your partner about cuckolding fantasies?

Cuckolding is a sexual practice and relationship dynamic in which a person, typically a man (called a "cuckold"), derives pleasure from the fact that his partner, often a woman (called a "cuckoldress"), has sexual intercourse with other people. This practice can include varying levels of involvement and awareness, and often involves an element of consensual humiliation, voyeurism, and power dynamics.

Origins and meaning

The term "cuckold" has ancient origins and derives from the Middle English "cokewold," which is related to the word "cuckoo," a bird known for laying its eggs in other birds' nests. In the sexual and relational context, modern cuckolding is a consensual fantasy and practice that has evolved and distanced itself from its original meaning, which implied non-consensual infidelity.

Elements of Cuckolding

Cuckolding can include a variety of elements, depending on the preferences and limits of the couple involved:

1.   **Voyeurism:** The "cuckold" partner may find it exciting to watch their partner have sexual relations with other people.

2.   **Consensual Humiliation:** Some people find excitement in the dynamic of consensual humiliation, where the cuckolded partner is teased or humiliated in a safe and consensual context.

3.   **Complicity and communication:** Open communication and complicity between partners are fundamental. Everyone must agree and be comfortable with the situation.

4.   **Fantasy and Reality:** Cuckolding can be experienced as a fantasy through conversations, sexting, or pornography, or it can be practiced in reality with actual sexual encounters.

Motivations and pleasure

The motivations behind cuckolding can vary greatly from person to person. Some possible reasons include:

Excitement from consensual infidelity: The idea of "sharing" one's partner can be extremely exciting for some people.

Power and control: The power dynamic and the role of submission can be key elements.

Self-Esteem and Inadequacy: Some people may find pleasure in facing and transforming feelings of inadequacy or insecurity.

Variety and novelty: Introducing a third person can add an element of variety and novelty to a couple's sex life.

As with all sexual practices, it is essential that all parties involved are aware of each other's limits, expectations, and desires. Establishing "safe words" and having a plan to stop the activity if someone feels uncomfortable is fundamental to ensuring the experience is safe and enjoyable for everyone.

Cuckolding is a complex sexual practice that can offer pleasure and satisfaction to those who find this dynamic exciting. The key to exploring cuckolding in a safe and consensual way is open and honest communication between partners, respect for limits, and a strong focus on mutual consent. As with any fantasy or sexual practice, it is important that all parties involved feel respected, listened to, and safe.

Talking to your partner about cuckolding fantasies

Talking to your partner about cuckolding fantasies can be a delicate conversation, but addressing it with sincerity and respect can open new possibilities in the relationship. The first step is to create an environment of open and non-judgmental communication. Choose a quiet and private moment where both of you feel relaxed and unhurried. It is important to be calm and clear, explaining that you want to talk about a sexual fantasy without any pressure or expectation.

When introducing the topic of cuckolding, it is essential to explain what it means to you and why it appeals to you. You might say, "Cuckolding is a fantasy that excites me because… (explain your reasons, such as the desire to see your partner's pleasure, the thrill of transgression, etc.). I know it might seem unusual, but I would like to understand with you if it is something we can explore safely and consensually."

It is equally important to be ready to listen to your partner and respect their reactions. They might be surprised, curious, or even concerned. Leave room for their questions and feelings, and respond with patience and sincerity. The key is to maintain an open dialogue and reassure your partner that their feelings are valid and as important as yours.

It may also be useful to discuss limits and concerns. Make sure your partner understands that there is no pressure to act immediately on this fantasy and that your relationship and their comfort are your absolute priority.

The most important thing is that both parties feel respected, heard, and safe while exploring new dimensions of their sexuality. The process of open and continuous communication can strengthen the bond between you, regardless of whether you decide to explore cuckolding or not.

How can one explore their bisexuality within a heterosexual relationship?

Exploring your bisexuality within a heterosexual relationship can be a complex but deeply enriching experience. The first fundamental step is personal reflection. Take the time to understand what being bisexual means to you and how you wish to explore this part of your identity. You may discover that you are primarily interested in exploring these fantasies on an emotional and mental level, or you may have a desire for physical experiences. Understanding your motivations and desires will help you communicate better with your partner.

Once you have reflected on your feelings, the next step is to talk openly with your partner. Listening carefully to your partner's reaction is essential. They may have questions, concerns, or strong feelings about your revelation. It's important to respect their feelings and respond with empathy and patience. Emphasize that your exploration of bisexuality does not diminish your love and commitment to them, but is a part of you that you wish to understand better.

If your partner is open to the idea, you could explore together how to integrate this aspect of your sexuality into your relationship. This could include discussing limits, boundaries, and safe ways to explore these new dynamics. Some couples find it helpful to participate in support groups or counseling with therapists specializing in sexuality to navigate these conversations.

In some cases, your partner may have difficulty understanding or accepting this aspect of your identity. It's important to give space and time to process this information and continue to communicate openly. If necessary, seeking the support of a therapist can help both of you navigate these feelings constructively.

Exploring your bisexuality does not necessarily mean acting on desires with other people. It can also mean reading, watching films, or simply discussing your fantasies openly. Every couple can find their unique way to integrate this exploration into their relationship.

Ultimately, the key is to remain empathetic towards your partner's feelings and navigate this journey of discovery together. With the right approach, exploring bisexuality can strengthen the connection and mutual understanding within the relationship.

Is it possible to have orgasms through mental stimulation alone?

Yes, it is possible to have orgasms through mental stimulation alone.

This phenomenon is known as a mental orgasm or orgasm without physical contact and can occur due to the power of imagination, sexual fantasies, and mental focus.

The brain is the most powerful and complex sexual organ in the human body. Many people find that they can achieve orgasm through intense erotic thoughts, vivid visualizations, and the release of endorphins and other neurotransmitters associated with pleasure. This process involves the ability to immerse oneself completely in one's fantasies and use breathing and relaxation techniques to intensify sensations.

Some techniques that can help achieve a mental orgasm include meditation and mindfulness. These practices help develop greater awareness of one's body and sensations, allowing for better focus on erotic images and thoughts. Some people also use tantra, which emphasizes the connection between mind and body and breath control to increase sexual arousal.

Autosuggestion and hypnosis can be other useful techniques. Some people can self-hypnotize or use guided recordings to enter a state of deep relaxation and concentration, which facilitates the experience of a mental orgasm.

For many people, mental stimulation can be combined with physical stimulation to intensify the orgasm experience. However, the ability to reach orgasm solely through the mind is a testament to the complex interaction between mind and body in human sexuality.

It is important to explore and discover what works best for you without judgment or pressure. The key is to be open to your own experiences and desires and allow the brain to play its central role in the experience of sexual pleasure.

Is it normal to desire sex with much younger or older people?

Yes, it is perfectly normal to desire sex with much younger or older people. Sexual and romantic attraction can vary greatly from person to person and can be influenced by a wide range of factors, including personal experiences, individual preferences, and relational dynamics.

Attraction to people of different ages can have different motivations. For example, some people may be attracted to the experience and maturity they find in older partners, appreciating the security, wisdom, and stability these relationships can offer. On the other hand, some may be attracted to the energy, freshness, and vitality of younger partners, finding in them a source of excitement and novelty.

It is important to emphasize that these attractions, like any other, must be managed with respect, consent, and awareness of the power dynamics that can exist in relationships with a significant age difference. When a relationship involves partners of different ages, it is crucial to ensure that both parties are consenting and have sufficient age and maturity to understand and manage the implications of their relationship.

Society may have different opinions regarding relationships with large age differences, often based on cultural and moral norms. However, as long as the relationship is based on mutual consent, there is nothing inherently wrong with desiring or having a relationship with someone of a very different age.

If you find yourself having these desires, it is useful to reflect on what attracts you to partners of different ages and consider how these desires align with your values and relational goals. Openly discussing your preferences and expectations with your partner (current or potential) can help build a healthy and respectful relationship.

Is it possible to have an orgasm through breast stimulation alone?

Yes, it is possible to have an orgasm through breast stimulation alone. The breasts are an erogenous zone for many people and, if stimulated adequately, can lead to a high level of sexual arousal and even orgasm. This is due to the presence of numerous nerve endings in the breasts and nipples, which, when stimulated, can send pleasure signals to the brain.

The ability to reach orgasm through breast stimulation varies from person to person. Some people may find it highly effective and pleasurable, while others may not achieve the same level of pleasure or reach orgasm this way. The body's response to breast stimulation depends on individual factors such as sensitivity, arousal, and personal preferences.

For many women, combining breast stimulation with other forms of sexual stimulation, such as clitoral or vaginal stimulation, can significantly increase pleasure and the likelihood of reaching orgasm.

Why do some men lose their erection during sex?

Losing an erection during sex is a phenomenon that can be caused by various physical and psychological factors. One of the most common reasons is performance anxiety, which can make a man feel pressured to "perform" well, creating a cycle of stress that makes it difficult to maintain an erection. General stress, depression, and other psychological conditions can also negatively affect erectile function.

On the physical level, health issues such as diabetes, cardiovascular diseases, and hormonal imbalances can compromise blood flow to the penis. Additionally, the use of alcohol and drugs, as well as some medications, can have negative effects on erection. Finally, relational problems or a lack of attraction can contribute to this situation. In any case, it is important to communicate openly with your partner and, if necessary, consult a healthcare professional to identify and treat the underlying causes.

Does frequent masturbation cause erectile dysfunction?

Frequent masturbation, in itself, does not cause erectile dysfunction (ED). However, there are some aspects to consider regarding how masturbation can temporarily influence sexual function and well-being:

1. **Temporary psychological and physical effects:**

   Temporary Desensitization: Frequent masturbation, especially if done with techniques that do not replicate the sensations of sex with a partner, could temporarily desensitize the nerves in the penis, making it more difficult to achieve or maintain an erection during intercourse. This desensitization is generally temporary and can resolve with a break from masturbation. **Habit to Certain Stimuli:** If a person becomes accustomed to a certain type of stimulation during masturbation, they may find it difficult to reach the same level of arousal during intercourse. This can create psychological difficulties, but it is not true erectile dysfunction.

2. **Mental health and stress:**

Performance Anxiety: Worrying about sexual performance can cause anxiety, which in turn can affect the ability to maintain an erection. This is not caused by masturbation but rather the psychological response to it.

Guilt or Shame: Feeling guilty or ashamed about masturbation can contribute to psychogenic erectile dysfunction.

3.   **Physical issues:**

Physical Trauma: Too vigorous masturbation can cause temporary irritation or damage to penile tissues, which could temporarily affect erectile function.

4.   **Positive effects of masturbation:**

Stress Relief: Masturbation can help reduce stress and anxiety, which are risk factors for erectile dysfunction.

Knowledge of One's Body: Masturbation helps better understand one's body and sexual responses, which can improve sexual function and communication with a partner.

5.   **Myths and reality:**

Popular Myths: There are many cultural myths and taboos about masturbation that can cause unfounded concerns. There is no scientific evidence that frequent masturbation causes long-term erectile dysfunction.

Practical advice

Vary Techniques: If frequent masturbation is negatively affecting your sexual life with a partner, it can be helpful to vary techniques and temporarily reduce the frequency.

Consult a Doctor: If you experience persistent erectile dysfunction, it is important to consult a doctor to rule out underlying medical causes and receive appropriate advice.

Balance Frequency: Maintain a balance in the frequency of masturbation, ensuring it does not interfere with your sexual life with a partner.

How can erectile dysfunction be overcome without medication?

Overcoming erectile dysfunction without medication is possible through a series of strategies aimed at improving physical and mental health. The first important step is to adopt a healthy lifestyle. Maintaining a balanced diet, rich in fruits, vegetables, whole grains, and lean proteins, can improve blood circulation and overall health, reducing the risk of erectile dysfunction. Regular physical exercise, such as walking, running, or yoga, can increase endurance, improve circulation, and reduce stress.

Reducing or eliminating alcohol consumption and quitting smoking are other crucial steps, as both habits can negatively affect erectile function. Weight control is also important, as obesity is a risk factor for erectile dysfunction.

Stress and anxiety management is equally fundamental. Relaxation techniques such as meditation, deep breathing, and mindfulness can help reduce stress and improve the quality of sexual life. Cognitivebehavioral therapy (CBT) can be useful for addressing performance anxiety or other psychological issues that contribute to erectile dysfunction.

Another important aspect is communication with your partner. Openly talking about your difficulties and concerns can reduce anxiety and improve the relationship. Couples therapy can be helpful for improving communication and addressing any relational problems that may affect sexual function.

Adopting specific techniques to improve erectile function can be useful. Pelvic floor exercises, known as Kegel exercises, can strengthen the muscles involved in erection. Additionally, taking the time to create a relaxed and pleasant atmosphere before sexual intercourse can help reduce anxiety and improve performance.

In summary, overcoming erectile dysfunction without medication requires a holistic approach involving lifestyle changes, stress management, and the adoption of specific techniques to improve sexual function. These changes can lead to significant and lasting improvements in the quality of sexual life.

Watching porn while in a relationship is not inherently wrong, but the issue is complex and depends greatly on the specific dynamics of each couple. The most important factor is open and honest communication between partners. Talking about your habits and preferences regarding pornography can help build a foundation of trust and mutual understanding. If both partners are aware of each other's habits and agree on what is acceptable, it can be less problematic.

The motivations behind consuming pornography are crucial. If used as a complement to the couple's sex life and not as a substitute, it may not be harmful. However, if it is used to avoid intimacy or address relationship problems, it could indicate a deeper issue that needs attention.

Pornography can also influence the perception of sexuality and the body, creating unrealistic expectations that could put pressure on one or both partners.

In some cases, excessive use of pornography can become a problem, interfering with daily life and relationships. If it becomes an addiction, it may be necessary to seek professional support to address the situation. It is essential to respect the feelings and boundaries of your partner. If one of you has difficulty accepting that the other watches porn, it is important to address the issue with empathy and seek a compromise that works for both.

In conclusion, there is no one-size-fits-all answer. Each couple must find a balance that works for both, through respect and mutual understanding.

How can vaginal dryness be addressed?

Here are some suggestions for addressing vaginal dryness in a natural and safe way:

Use water-based or silicone-based vaginal lubricants without preservatives. These can help temporarily alleviate dryness during intercourse.

Increase stimulation and pleasure before sexual intercourse to promote better natural lubrication.

Take supplements based on soy isoflavones or other plant sources of estrogen, after consulting with a doctor, as they can improve lubrication.

Massage the perineal area with natural oils such as coconut oil or sweet almond oil to hydrate the skin.

Avoid harsh intimate cleansers
and soaps that can alter vaginal pH.
Reduce stress factors that can
interfere with normal lubrication.

If the problem persists, it is advisable to consult a gynecologist to identify the underlying causes and rule out medical conditions such as hormonal deficiencies, medication side effects, or health problems.

How can pain during sex be addressed?

Addressing pain during sex requires a delicate and multifaceted approach, understanding both physical and emotional aspects. First of all, it is essential to communicate openly with your partner about the pain. This helps create an environment of understanding and support. Additionally, it is important to never force sexual activities and respect your body's limits.

Pain during sex can have many causes, including physical problems such as infections, vaginal dryness, or medical conditions like endometriosis. In these cases, consulting a doctor is essential to receive a diagnosis and appropriate treatment. Using lubricants can help reduce friction and improve comfort during intercourse.

Preparation is also crucial: taking time for foreplay can help relax the muscles and increase natural lubrication. If the pain is related to psychological or emotional issues, such as anxiety or stress, talking to a therapist specializing in sexology can be helpful.

Modifying sexual positions can reduce pain. Some positions may put less pressure on sensitive or problematic areas of the body. Finally, listening to your body and taking breaks when necessary helps avoid worsening the pain and makes the sexual experience more pleasant and safe.

Is it possible to have a satisfying sex life without penetration?

Yes, it is absolutely possible to have a fulfilling and satisfying sex life without vaginal or anal penetration. There are many other forms of intimacy, pleasure, and stimulation that a couple can explore:

Oral Sex: Both fellatio and cunnilingus can easily lead to orgasm and create an intense physical connection.

Manual Stimulation: Using hands, fingers, and massage on the genitals and the entire body can be extremely pleasurable.

Role-Playing/Seduction: Desire and excitement can be fueled through spicy conversations, the use of sex toys, lingerie, etc.

Nipple Stimulation: Many people find great pleasure in having their nipples licked, bitten, and gently massaged.

Intergenital Friction: Rubbing the genitals can create intense orgasmic sensations without penetration.

Shared Kinks and Fetishes: For some couples, activities like bondage, dominance/submission create much excitement.

The important thing is to keep an open mind, communicate openly about your desires, and respect your partner's limits. With creativity and commitment, it is possible to have a full sexual life without necessarily involving penetration.

How can sex be made safe without compromising pleasure?

Here are some tips to make sexual activity safer without compromising pleasure:

1.   **Always use male or female condoms** to protect against sexually transmitted infections (STIs) and unwanted pregnancies. Choose good quality condoms of different sizes/textures to find the most comfortable ones.

2.   **Communicate openly with your partner** about desires, limits, and both partners' health status. Be honest and avoid unnecessary risks.

3.   **Know the anatomy and erogenous zones** of your own body and your partner's body to maximize pleasure safely.

4.   **Experiment with positions, lubricants, and sex toys** that allow for pleasure without penetration if necessary.

5.   **Get regular STI screenings** if you have multiple occasional partners.

6.   **Learn and practice safe oral sex** by using dental dams or condoms.

7.   **Maintain excellent intimate hygiene** for both partners before engaging in sexual activity.

8.   **Agree on clear boundaries and rules** if you want to try practices like bondage or BDSM.

The goal is to experiment freely and creatively while taking appropriate precautions to protect the health and safety of both partners. Pleasure is maximized when both partners feel protected and respected.

Is it normal for libido to decrease during pregnancy?

Yes, it is absolutely normal for libido (sexual desire) to fluctuate during pregnancy. Here are some factors that can influence a decrease in desire during this period:

1.   **Hormonal changes** - Levels of estrogen and progesterone vary significantly, affecting arousal and lubrication.

2.   **Fatigue and nausea** - Especially in the first months, many women feel more tired and have nausea that can reduce interest in sexual activity.

3.   **Worries/Anxieties** - Concerns about the pregnancy, body changes, and risks can inhibit desire.

4.   **Physical pains and discomforts** - Back pain, breast sensitivity, and constipation can be anti-erotic factors.

5.   **Embarrassment about body changes** - Some women feel uncomfortable with their new body image.

However, not all women experience a decrease in libido during pregnancy. For some, desire may even increase, especially in the second trimester when initial side effects decrease.

The important thing is not to force yourself and to listen to your feelings. Communicate openly with your partner and find forms of intimacy other than full intercourse. After childbirth, hormone levels will gradually rebalance.

How can the decrease in sexual desire postpartum be addressed?

A decrease in sexual desire after childbirth is a very common and understandable phenomenon for several reasons. Firstly, the new mother's body has just gone through an extremely demanding physical experience such as childbirth, which requires a period of recovery and rest. This is compounded by drastic hormonal changes, with a drop in estrogen and testosterone levels that directly influence libido. Constant fatigue due to sleepless nights caring for the newborn is another factor that can negatively impact sexual desire.

Additionally, psychological and emotional factors such as anxiety, stress, low self-esteem related to body changes, or simply the fatigue of managing new parental responsibilities can exist. However, it is important for both partners to understand that this is a transitional phase and that with patience, open communication, and complicity, sexual desire can gradually return to previous levels. Taking time for self-care, relaxation, and strengthening the couple's bond, as well as physical intimacy through cuddles, massages, and other forms of non-sexual contact, can help rekindle passion when you feel ready again.

Sex after childbirth: When is it safe to resume?

Resuming sexual activity after childbirth is an important topic that involves physical, emotional, and relational aspects. It is crucial to understand that every woman and every childbirth is unique, so the timing can vary. However, there are some general guidelines and considerations that can help determine when it is safe to resume sexual activity after childbirth.

Physical considerations

1. **Recovery time:** Doctors usually recommend waiting at least 6 weeks after a vaginal delivery before resuming sexual activity. This period allows the body to heal, particularly the uterus, cervix, and any tears or incisions (such as an episiotomy). In the case of a cesarean delivery, more time may be needed for the surgical wound to heal.

2. **Postpartum bleeding:** After childbirth, it is common to have vaginal bleeding (lochia) that can last up to 6 weeks. It is advisable to wait until this bleeding significantly decreases to reduce the risk of infections.

3.   **Pain and Discomfort:** Many women may experience pain or discomfort during the first sexual encounters after childbirth. This may be due to tears, stitches, vaginal dryness, or other physiological changes. It is important to listen to your body and not force anything.

Emotional considerations

1.   **Stress and fatigue:** The birth of a child brings significant changes to a couple's life, which can be accompanied by stress and lack of sleep. These factors can influence sexual desire and the energy available for intimacy.

2.   **Body image:** Some women may feel insecure about their bodies after childbirth, which can affect their willingness to resume sexual activity.

3.   **Emotional connection:** It is important for both partners to feel ready and have open communication about their needs and desires. The resumption of intimacy should be a gradual and consensual process.

Practical tips

- **Lubricants:** Using water-based lubricants can help reduce discomfort caused by vaginal dryness, which is common after childbirth.

- **Comfortable positions:** Experiment with different sexual positions to find those that are most comfortable and least painful.

- **Consult a doctor:** If there are doubts or persistent problems, it is always best to consult a doctor or gynecologist. They can provide personalized advice based on the specific situation.

Is sex during breastfeeding safe?

Sex during breastfeeding is generally safe, but there are some physical and emotional considerations to keep in mind. Here is a detailed overview of this topic:

Physical considerations

Hormonal changes: During breastfeeding, a woman's body produces high levels of prolactin and oxytocin. Prolactin is responsible for milk production and can reduce sexual desire. Oxytocin, released during breastfeeding and orgasm, promotes bonding between mother and child but can also influence mood and interest in sex.

Vaginal lubrication: High levels of prolactin can reduce estrogen levels, leading to vaginal dryness. This can make sexual intercourse less comfortable or even painful. Using a water-based lubricant can help mitigate this problem.

Pain and discomfort: After childbirth, there may be residual pain, especially if there were tears, an episiotomy, or a cesarean section. It is important to wait until the body has completely healed before resuming sexual activity. Additionally, breastfeeding can cause nipple and breast pain, which may be more sensitive during sexual activity.

Emotional considerations

Fatigue and stress: Breastfeeding, along with caring for a newborn, can be physically and emotionally exhausting. Lack of sleep and changes in daily routines can affect desire and energy for sex.

Changes in body image: Women may feel insecure about changes in their postpartum body. Partner support and understanding are crucial during this period.

Precautions to take

Contraception: Although breastfeeding can reduce fertility and delay the return of the menstrual cycle (a phenomenon known as lactational amenorrhea), it is not a completely reliable contraceptive method. It is possible to ovulate before the return of menstruation, so it is important to discuss safe contraceptive options with a doctor during breastfeeding.

Practical tips

1.   **Lubrication:** Use water-based lubricants to reduce discomfort due to vaginal dryness.

2.   **Timing:** Choose moments when both partners feel relaxed and not too tired to improve the experience.

3.   **Comfortable positions:** Experiment with sexual positions that do not put pressure on the breasts and are comfortable for both partners.

4.   **Gradual pace:** Resume sexual activity gradually, listening to your body and respecting your limits.

How can one talk about sex with children in an open and honest way?

Talking about sex with children is a fundamental aspect of sexual education and their healthy development. Here are some tips on how to approach this topic in an open and honest way:

1. **Start early:** It's never too early to start talking about sex. Adjust the language and information to the child's age. For younger children, start with the correct names of body parts and a basic understanding of reproduction.

2. **Create a trusting environment:** Let your children know they can ask you anything without fear of being judged or punished. Show them you are available to talk about any topic.

3. **Use clear and simple language:** Avoid euphemisms and confusing terms. Use age-appropriate language that is clear and precise. Explain concepts in a simple and direct way.

4. **Be honest:** If you don't know the answer to a question, admit it and propose to look for the information together. Being honest builds trust and shows that learning is a continuous process.

5.   **Respect Their Curiosity:** Answer questions when they are asked. Don't avoid the topic or delay the answers. Their curiosity is natural and should be respected.

6.   **Approach the topic progressively:** Introduce more complex information as your children grow. The conversation about sexual education should be continuous and adapt to their level of development.

7.   **Talk about values and relationships:** Beyond the physical aspects of sex, discuss emotions, relationships, and personal values. Talk about respect, consent, and responsibility in intimate relationships.

8.   **Use educational resources:** Books, educational videos, and articles can be helpful tools. Ensure the resources are age-appropriate and suitable for your children's maturity.

9.   **Model healthy behavior:** Your children learn by observing your behavior. Show respect for yourself and others, and practice open and honest communication in your relationships.

10. **Stay available:** Let your children know you are always available to talk, not just during a scheduled "big conversation." Continuous availability is important for maintaining open communication.

Promoting open and honest sexual education helps children develop a healthy and secure view of sexuality and relationships.

What are the best sex toys for couples?

Here are some of the best and most common sex toys that couples can use to enrich their intimate life:

Vibrators: There are models of various shapes, sizes, and power levels to stimulate both female genitals and other erogenous zones of both partners.

Vibrating Penis Rings: They can prolong the erection and stimulate both partners during penetration.

Lubricants: Both water-based and silicone-based, they facilitate friction and comfortable penetration, even during foreplay.

Light Bondage: Handcuffs, blindfolds, and soft ropes can add a playful touch of submission for those who like to experiment.

Butt Plugs and Anal Vibrators: For those who want to explore anal pleasure gradually and safely.

Couple's Massagers: Ideal for sensual full-body massage before sexual activity.

Sex Pillows and Cushions: They facilitate certain positions and can make intercourse more comfortable.

The important thing is to choose quality toys made of safe and non-toxic materials.

Is it possible to have an active and satisfying sex life in old age?

Yes, it is absolutely possible to have an active and satisfying sex life even in old age. Here are some important factors to consider:

1.   **Accept normal physical changes with an open mind:** Age-related sexual dysfunctions they must be accepted with open-mindedness, without precluding pleasure and intimacy. They may simply require a little more care.

2.   **Age-related sexual dysfunctions** (such as erectile difficulties or vaginal dryness) can be addressed and managed with lubricants, medications, stimulators, and specific therapies.

3.   **Maintain a healthy Lifestyle:** Regular physical activity, a balanced diet, and stress management can improve desire and sexual performance.

4.   **Open communication with the partner:** Discuss new needs, fantasies, and desires for a satisfying understanding.

5.   **Explore different forms of intimacy:** Oral sex, mutual masturbation, and manual stimulation are excellent alternatives to complete sexual intercourse.

6.   **Prolong foreplay:** Sensual massage and creating a relaxing atmosphere can increase excitement.

7.   **Keep an open mind and curiosity:** Trying new positions, places, or situations can rekindle desire.

With the right open-mindedness, fulfilling physical intimacy does not necessarily have an age limit.

Creativity and acceptance of changes are the main keys.

Is it normal to never have experienced an orgasm?

It is entirely normal and quite common to never have experienced an orgasm, especially for some women. The inability to reach orgasm, called anorgasmia, can have various physical, psychological, or combined causes.

From a physical standpoint, factors such as hormonal issues, side effects of medications, previous surgeries, or simply a lack of knowledge about one's own anatomy and erogenous zones can hinder the achievement of orgasm.

Similarly, psychological factors such as stress, anxiety, relationship problems, past traumas, or even the lack of adequate sexual education can inhibit the mental relaxation necessary to let go and experience orgasmic pleasure.

The important thing is not to develop excessive guilt or frustration. With patience, open communication with your partner, and possibly the support of a qualified sex therapist, you can explore and understand the specific obstacles and then work on the most effective strategies to adopt, such as meditation, erotic games, using lubricants or stimulators.

Remember that orgasm is not the only measure of a fulfilling sexual experience. Pleasure can be achieved in many other forms through intimacy, complicity, and emotional connection with your partner. The important thing is to relax and not force things.

How can one address sexual trauma and regain a healthy sex life?

Addressing sexual trauma and regaining a healthy sex life is a delicate process that requires time, patience, and adequate support. Here are some steps that can help:

1. **Acknowledge the trauma**

   Accept your feelings: It is normal to feel a range of emotions such as anger, sadness, confusion, or fear. Recognizing and accepting these feelings is the first step towards healing.

   Avoid self-blame: Sexual trauma is the fault of the perpetrator, not the victim. It is important to remember that you are not responsible for the abuse you suffered.

2. **Seek professional support**

   Specialized Therapist: Consulting a therapist specialized in sexual trauma can offer targeted and professional support. Therapy may include various methodologies such as cognitivebehavioral therapy (CBT), EMDR (Eye Movement Desensitization and Reprocessing), or somatic therapy.

Support groups: Participating in support groups for victims of sexual trauma can help you feel less alone and share experiences with those who have gone through similar situations.

3.   **Education and awareness**

Know your rights: Being informed about your rights and the resources available can provide a sense of empowerment.

Sexual Education: Learning more about sexuality, your limits, and desires can help you regain control over your sexual life.

4.   **Work on the relationship with your body**

Mindfulness practices: Activities like meditation, yoga, and mindfulness can help you reconnect with your body in a safe and positive way.

Self-care: Taking care of your body through rest, healthy eating, and physical exercise can contribute to overall well-being.

5.   **Start gradually**

Respect your own pace: There is no rush to return to an active sex life. It is important to respect your own pace and move forward only when you feel ready.

Individual Exploration: Masturbation can be a safe way to explore your body and understand what you find pleasurable without the pressure of a partner.

6.   **Communication with your partner**

Be open and honest: Share your experiences, limits, and needs with your partner. An understanding and patient partner can make a big difference.

Establish clear boundaries: Discuss and establish clear boundaries about what is acceptable and what is not during intimacy.

7.   **Positive experiences**

Create new experiences: Working to build positive and consensual sexual experiences can help replace traumatic memories with more pleasant and reassuring ones.

Sex toys and experimentation: If you feel comfortable, using sex toys or exploring new practices can help you rediscover pleasure in a safe way.

8.   **Continuous support**

Ongoing Therapy: Continuing to see a therapist or participating in support groups even after starting to feel better can provide a safety net and continuous help.

Recognize progress: Celebrating small progress and recognizing the efforts made can help maintain motivation and a sense of hope.

Recovery from sexual trauma is an individual and unique journey for each person. It is important to be kind to yourself and seek the necessary support to regain a healthy and satisfying sexual life.

What are the signs of sexual addiction and how can it be addressed?

Sexual addiction, or hypersexuality, is a condition where a person's sexual behavior becomes compulsive and negatively interferes with daily life, relationships, and overall well-being. Here are the common signs of sexual addiction and how to address it:

Signs of sexual addiction

1. **Constant Preoccupation with Sex:**

    Persistent sexual thoughts that distract from daily activities and work tasks.

2. **Loss of control:**

    Inability to limit or stop sexual behaviors despite repeated attempts.

3. **Compulsive sexual activity:**

    Engagement in multiple sexual activities, including pornography, masturbation, casual sex, excessive attendance at sex-themed venues.

4. **Using sex to manage emotions:**

Resorting to sex as a way to cope with stress, loneliness, sadness, or anxiety.

5.   **Negative Consequences:**

Experiencing relationship problems, job loss, financial issues, or legal problems due to sexual behavior.

6.   **Feeling shame and guilt:**

Feeling guilty or ashamed of one's sexual behavior but continuing to engage in it nonetheless.

7.   **Social withdrawal:**

Avoiding social interactions and non-sexual activities because of sexual behavior.

How to Address Sexual Addiction

1.   **Acknowledge the problem:**

The first step is admitting you have a problem. Awareness is crucial for starting the recovery process.

2.   **Seek professional support:**

Individual Therapy: A therapist specialized in sexual addictions can help identify underlying causes and develop strategies to manage the behavior.

Group Therapy: Participating in support groups for people with sexual addictions can provide a safe environment to share experiences and receive support.

3.   **Education and awareness:**

Learn about sexual addiction, its effects, and recovery strategies. Knowledge helps better understand your condition.

4.   **Establish clear boundaries:**

Define clear limits for sexual behavior and commit to adhering to them. This may include avoiding triggers like pornography or risky situations.

5.   **Manage stress and emotions:**

Learn stress management techniques such as meditation, yoga, physical exercise, and cognitivebehavioral therapy (CBT) to cope with emotions without resorting to sex.

6.   **Build a support network:**

Talk to friends, family, or partners who can offer emotional support and understanding during the recovery journey.

7.   **Avoid triggers:**

Identify and avoid situations, places, or people that may trigger compulsive behavior.

8. **Develop new habits and interests:**

Cultivate hobbies and activities that are not related to sex to fill time and energy with positive and constructive experiences.

9. **Monitor progress:**

Keep a journal to monitor progress, challenges, and victories in the recovery journey. This can help maintain motivation and identify behavior patterns.

10. **Be patient with yourself:**

Recovery from addiction is a long and challenging process. It is important to be kind to yourself and recognize that change takes time.

Addressing sexual addiction requires commitment and the right support, but with determination and professional help, it is possible to recover and build a healthy and balanced sexual life.

Do vibrators reduce sensitivity?

No, vibrators do not permanently reduce sexual sensitivity. However, some people may experience temporary numbness or decreased sensitivity if they use a vibrator on a very high setting for a prolonged period. This reduction in sensitivity is usually temporary and typically resolves quickly after discontinuing vibrator use.

It is important to listen to your body and take breaks if you feel numbness or decreased sensitivity. Using the vibrator at different intensity settings and varying the type of stimulation can help avoid any temporary discomfort.

Using vibrators can also have many positive benefits, such as increasing awareness of your body and pleasure, improving the quality of orgasms, and promoting greater sexual exploration. The key is to use vibrators in a way that is enjoyable and comfortable for you.

Is the withdrawal method an effective contraceptive?

No, the withdrawal method (or "pull-out method") is not an effective contraceptive method. This method involves withdrawing the penis from the vagina before ejaculation to prevent sperm from coming into contact with the egg. However, it has several issues that significantly reduce its effectiveness:

1. **Pre-ejaculatory Fluid:** Before ejaculation, a man may release pre-ejaculatory fluid (pre-cum) that can contain sperm and thus can cause pregnancy.

2. **Timing and Control:** It requires great control and timing from the man, which can be difficult to manage during moments of high sexual excitement.

3. **Human Error:** Even with perfect control, there is always the risk of human error. Even a small amount of sperm can be enough to cause pregnancy.

According to some studies, the withdrawal method has a failure rate of 22% with typical use, meaning that 22 out of 100 women who use this method for a year will become pregnant.

For more reliable contraception, it is advisable to use methods such as condoms, birth control pills, intrauterine devices (IUDs), or other approved contraceptive methods. These methods are not only more effective at preventing pregnancy, but some, like condoms, also offer protection against sexually transmitted infections (STIs).

Does Viagra cause heart attacks?

No, Viagra (sildenafil) does not cause heart attacks if used correctly and under medical supervision. Viagra is an approved medication for treating erectile dysfunction and works by increasing blood flow to the penis to help maintain an erection. However, there are some important considerations to keep in mind:

1.   **Pre-existing health conditions:** Viagra can be dangerous for men with certain health conditions, such as severe cardiovascular diseases, very low blood pressure, or those taking nitrate-based medications for heart problems. In these cases, using Viagra can increase the risk of cardiac complications.

2.   **Interaction with other medications:** Viagra can interact with some medications, particularly nitrates, causing a dangerous drop in blood pressure. It is essential to inform your doctor of all medications you are taking before starting Viagra treatment.

3.   **Side effects:** While it does not cause heart attacks, Viagra can have side effects such as headaches, flushing, indigestion, visual disturbances, and, in rare cases, chest pain. If you experience chest pain or symptoms similar to those of a

heart attack while using Viagra, it is important to seek immediate medical assistance.

4.   **Proper use:** Viagra should be taken according to the doctor's instructions. Do not exceed the prescribed dose or use it more frequently than recommended.

In general, for healthy men without medical contraindications, Viagra is safe and does not increase the risk of a heart attack. It is always important to discuss with a doctor to evaluate whether Viagra is a safe and appropriate option for your specific situation.

Can sex cause heart attacks?

Sex can rarely cause heart attacks, but for most people, it is a safe and beneficial activity for health. Here are some important considerations:

Risk of heart attack during sex

1.   **General population:**

For healthy people, the risk of having a heart attack during sex is extremely low. Sex is a form of moderate physical activity that can temporarily increase heart rate and blood pressure, but not enough to cause heart problems in most individuals.

2.   **People with heart problems:**

For those with pre-existing heart diseases, such as a history of heart attacks, angina, or heart failure, the risk may be slightly higher. However, even in these cases, the risk is relatively low if the person is stabilized and follows the doctor's recommendations.

Studies and data

Research on sex safety:

Studies have shown that less than 1% of heart attacks occur during sexual activity. For example, research from St. George's University of London found that only 0.2% of heart attack deaths occur during sex.

Another study demonstrated that sex represents an increased risk of heart attack by about 2.5 times compared to rest, but since the baseline risk is very low, the relative increase is still insignificant for most people.

Benefits of sex

— Cardiovascular Health:

Regular sex can improve cardiovascular health, lower blood pressure, and reduce stress. These overall benefits can actually reduce the long-term risk of heart problems.

— Hormones and Well-being:

Sexual activity releases endorphins and oxytocin, which improve mood and well-being, reducing stress, which is a risk factor for heart disease.

Precautions for people at risk

1. **Consult a doctor:**

Those with heart problems should consult their doctor to assess the safety of sexual activity. The doctor can provide specific advice based on the patient's individual condition.

2.   Modify activity:

If you have health problems, you can take steps to make sex safer, such as choosing less strenuous positions, avoiding sex immediately after a heavy meal, and recognizing your physical limits.

3.   Monitor symptoms:

Pay attention to symptoms such as chest pain, difficulty breathing, or irregular heartbeat. If they occur, it is important to stop and seek medical assistance.

In conclusion, for most people, sex is a safe and beneficial activity for health. The risk of heart attack during sex is very low, even for those with pre-existing heart conditions, as long as they follow medical recommendations and take appropriate precautions.

Does sex help you lose weight?

Sex can contribute to burning calories, but it is not sufficient on its own to cause significant weight loss. Here are some key points to consider:

1.   **Calories burned during sex:** Sexual activity burns calories, but the exact amount depends on various factors such as the intensity and duration of the act. On average, a sexual encounter lasting 25-30 minutes can burn approximately 100-150 calories for men and slightly less for women.

2.   **Comparison with other physical activities:** Sex burns fewer calories compared to many other forms of exercise. For instance, running, swimming, or doing aerobic workouts can burn many more calories in a similar amount of time.

3.   **Physical benefits of sex:** Although it is not a substitute for regular exercise, sex offers various health benefits, including improved circulation, a stronger immune system, and stress reduction.

4.   **Healthy lifestyle:** For significant weight loss, a more comprehensive approach is necessary, including a balanced diet and a regular exercise program. Sex can be part of a

healthy lifestyle, but it should not be the only strategy for losing weight.

5.   **Other benefits:** Regular sex can improve mood, reduce anxiety, and enhance the emotional bond with your partner, all of which contribute to overall better well-being.

In conclusion, while sex can help burn some calories, it is not sufficient alone for significant weight loss. Combining sexual activity with a healthy diet and regular physical exercise is the best way to achieve and maintain a healthy weight.

Does abstinence improve sperm quality?

Sexual abstinence can influence sperm quality, but not necessarily in a positive way. The relationship between abstinence and sperm quality is complex and depends on the duration of abstinence and the specific characteristics of the sperm being considered. Here is a more detailed overview:

Short periods of abstinence

Semen Volume: A few days of abstinence can increase ejaculate volume.

Sperm Count: Short-term abstinence (2-7 days) can increase the number of sperm per ejaculate, which can be useful for some assisted fertilization techniques.

Long periods of abstinence

Sperm Motility: Prolonged abstinence (more than 7 days) can reduce sperm motility, meaning their ability to swim effectively towards the egg.

Sperm Morphology: The shape and structure of sperm can also deteriorate with prolonged abstinence, affecting their ability to fertilize the egg.

DNA Damage: Prolonged abstinence can increase DNA fragmentation in sperm, reducing the genetic quality of the sperm.

Optimization for fertility

Ideal frequency: For men with fertility issues, an interval of 2-3 days of abstinence is often recommended to optimize both the number and quality of sperm.

Regular ejaculations: To maintain good sperm quality, regular ejaculations are generally preferable. Studies have shown that ejaculating every 2-3 days can help keep sperm in optimal condition.

Additional factors

Lifestyle and Diet: A healthy diet, regular physical exercise, avoiding smoking and alcohol, and reducing stress can significantly impact sperm quality.

Hydration: Drinking plenty of water can help maintain an adequate ejaculate volume and improve sperm quality.

Supplements: Some supplements, such as zinc, selenium, vitamin E, and antioxidants, can improve sperm quality.

Research and evidence

Clinical Studies: Some studies have shown that daily ejaculation for 7 days can improve sperm DNA quality, reducing DNA fragmentation and improving overall sperm health.

Individual Variability: The response to abstinence can vary between individuals. Therefore, men seeking to improve their fertility should consult a doctor or fertility specialist for personalized advice.

Do sexual positions influence the probability of conception?

Sexual positions can impact the probability of conception, although their influence is not as significant as other factors such as individual fertility, timing, and reproductive health. Here is a detailed overview of how sexual positions can influence the likelihood of conception:

Sexual positions and conception

1.	**Missionary Position (Man on Top):** This is one of the most recommended positions for conception because it allows for deep penetration, bringing the sperm closer to the cervix. Gravity can help the sperm reach the uterus more easily.

2.	**Doggy Style Position:** This position, with the woman on all fours and the man behind, allows for deep penetration and can bring the sperm closer to the cervix. Some research suggests that this position may be useful for women with a retroverted uterus (a uterus tilted backward).

3.	**Side-Lying Position (Spooning):** This position is less common but can be useful because it is comfortable and allows for adequate penetration. It is relaxing and can help the woman relax, reducing stress, which can be beneficial for conception.

Key factors to consider

1. **Timing:** The most important factor for conception is the timing of sexual intercourse in relation to the woman's ovulation cycle. Ovulation typically occurs in the middle of the menstrual cycle, and the most fertile days are those that precede and follow ovulation.

2. **Sperm Quality:** Sperm quality plays a crucial role in fertility. Healthy lifestyle habits such as a balanced diet, regular physical exercise, avoiding smoking, and limiting alcohol use can improve sperm quality.

3. **Reproductive Health:** The overall reproductive health of both partners is fundamental. Conditions such as endometriosis, sexually transmitted infections (STIs), and ovulation problems can affect fertility.

Additional practical tips

1. **Lying Down After Sex:** Some experts recommend lying down for 10-15 minutes after sexual intercourse to help the sperm reach the cervix. While there is no definitive scientific proof to support this practice, many couples find it useful.

2.   **Avoid Lubricants:** Some lubricants can negatively affect sperm motility. It is best to avoid them or use lubricants specifically formulated not to harm sperm.

3.   **Reduce Stress:** Stress can negatively affect fertility in both men and women. Relaxation techniques such as yoga, meditation, and other relaxing activities can be beneficial.

Can sex cause urinary tract infections?

Yes, sex can increase the risk of developing urinary tract infections (UTIs), especially in women. This correlation is due to various anatomical and behavioral factors. Here is a detailed explanation of how sex can cause urinary tract infections and how to prevent these infections:

How sex can cause urinary tract infections

1.   **Female Anatomy:** The female urethra is relatively short and located close to the anus and vagina. During sexual activity, bacteria present in the anal and vaginal areas can be pushed towards the urethra, increasing the risk of infection.

2.   **Bacteria and Friction:** Sexual activity can cause friction that facilitates the entry of bacteria into the urethra. The most common bacteria associated with UTIs is Escherichia coli (E. coli), normally present in the intestine.

3.   **Use of Diaphragms and Spermicides:** The use of certain contraceptives, such as diaphragms and spermicides, can alter the balance of bacteria in the vaginal area and increase the risk of UTIs.

4.	**Consecutive Anal and Vaginal Sex:** Switching from anal to vaginal sex without proper hygiene can transfer fecal bacteria to the urethra.

Symptoms of urinary tract infections

Common symptoms of a urinary tract infection include:

A burning sensation during urination

Frequent and urgent need to urinate, often with the emission of small amounts of urine

Cloudy urine or urine with a strong odor

Pain or pressure in the lower abdomen or pelvic area

In some cases, fever and lower back pain, which can indicate a more serious kidney infection

Preventing sex-related urinary tract infections

Here are some strategies to reduce the risk of developing UTIs after sexual activity:

1.	**Urinate Before and After Sex:** Urinating before and immediately after sex can help flush out bacteria that may have entered the urethra during sexual activity.

2.	**Good Hygiene:** Wash the genital area before and after sex to reduce the amount of bacteria present.

3.   **Drink Plenty of Water:** Maintaining good hydration helps produce more urine, which can help flush out bacteria from the urethra.

4.   **Avoid Diaphragms and Spermicides:** If prone to UTIs, it may be useful to discuss the use of alternative contraceptive methods with your doctor.

5.   **Breathable Clothing:** Wear cotton underwear and avoid tight clothing to reduce moisture and bacterial growth in the genital area.

Is sex in water safe?

Sex in water, such as in a pool, bathtub, sea, or lake, can be exciting but has safety and hygiene considerations. Here are key points to ensure a safe experience:

Safety and hygiene considerations

1.   Infections and Irritations

Bacteria and Chemicals: Water in pools and hot tubs can contain bacteria and chemicals like chlorine, which may cause irritation or infections. Seawater can also have bacteria.

Natural Lubrication: Water can wash away natural lubrication, increasing the risk of friction and irritation, leading to micro-injuries that facilitate infections.

Urinary Tract Infections (UTIs): Women are particularly susceptible to UTIs if bacteria enter the urethra during sex in water.

2. Contraception and Protection

Condom Efficacy: Water, especially with chlorine or salt, can compromise condom effectiveness, causing slippage or breakage, reducing protection against STIs and unwanted pregnancies.

Spermicides: Spermicides may be less effective in water, increasing pregnancy risk.

Practical safety tips

1. Hygiene and Infection Prevention

Clean Water: Ensure water is clean and free of harmful bacteria. Avoid stagnant or potentially contaminated water.

Shower Before and After: Showering before and after sex can reduce infection risk. Use antibacterial soap.

Lubricant: Use a water-resistant silicone-based lubricant to reduce friction and irritation.

2. Protection and Contraception

Quality Condoms: Use high-quality condoms and ensure they are securely fastened. Change condoms if necessary.

Additional Contraceptives: Consider additional or alternative contraceptive methods like birth control pills, IUDs, or vaginal rings.

Can sex cause allergies?

Yes, sex can cause allergic reactions, though they are relatively rare. Potential causes include allergies to condom materials and seminal fluid. Here's how to manage them:

Condom Material Allergies

1. **Latex:** Common symptoms include itching, redness, swelling, and hives in the genital area. Severe cases can involve respiratory issues and anaphylaxis.

2. **Alternatives:** Use condoms made from materials like polyurethane or polyisoprene if allergic to latex.

Lubricants and Intimate Products Allergies

1. **Chemical Ingredients:** Some lubricants, gels, and intimate products contain chemicals, fragrances, or preservatives that can cause allergic reactions or irritation.

2. **Natural Products:** Use natural, fragrance-free lubricants and products to reduce allergy risk.

Seminal Fluid Allergies

1. **Semen Allergy:** Rare but possible, causing burning, itching, and swelling in the vaginal area after intercourse.

Severe cases can cause systemic symptoms like hives and anaphylaxis.

2. **Diagnosis and Treatment:** Specific allergy tests can diagnose this condition. Treatment may involve using condoms to prevent contact or gradual desensitization under medical supervision.

Prevention and Management

1. **Identify Allergens:** If you suspect a sex-related allergy, identify the specific cause through allergy tests and consultations with a doctor.

2. **Alternative Products:** Use latex-free condoms, natural lubricants, and hypoallergenic skincare products.

3. **Communication:** Discuss allergies and preventive measures with your partner for a safe and enjoyable sexual life.

4. **Medical Consultation:** See an allergist or specialized doctor for an accurate diagnosis and allergy management plan.

Can sex influence the menstrual cycle?

Yes, sex can influence the menstrual cycle in various ways, which vary from person to person.

Positive Effects of Sex on the Menstrual Cycle

1.   **Cycle Regulation:** Regular sexual activity can help regulate the menstrual cycle. Orgasms release endorphins, reducing stress and balancing hormones, contributing to a more regular cycle.

2.   **Cramp Relief:** Sex can alleviate menstrual cramps. Orgasms cause uterine contractions that release prostaglandins, which help relieve menstrual pain. Endorphin release during orgasm acts as a natural painkiller.

Negative Effects of Sex on the Menstrual Cycle

1.   **Temporary Changes:** Some women may experience temporary changes in their cycle due to sex, such as light spotting or intermenstrual bleeding, especially if the cervix is irritated.

2.   **Stress and Anxiety:** If sex is associated with stress or anxiety, it can negatively impact the menstrual cycle. Stress can alter hormone levels and affect cycle regularity.

Considerations for Cycle Changes

1.   **Pregnancy:** A significant change in the menstrual cycle due to sex is the possibility of pregnancy. Missing a period is often the first sign of pregnancy. If there is a delay and unprotected sex has occurred, a pregnancy test is important.

2.   **Infections:** Sexually transmitted infections (STIs) can affect the menstrual cycle. For example, chlamydia and gonorrhea can cause abnormal bleeding. If an infection is suspected, consult a doctor.

Tips for Managing the Effects of Sex on the Menstrual Cycle

1.   **Monitor the Cycle:** Keeping track of the menstrual cycle can help identify any changes related to sexual activity. Cycle tracking apps can be useful for this purpose.

2.   **Communicate with the Partner:** Openly discussing how sexual activity affects the menstrual cycle can help find solutions that improve both partners' comfort and well-being.

3.   **Consult a Doctor:** If significant or concerning changes in the menstrual cycle are noticed, it is advisable to consult a doctor to rule out any underlying conditions.

Can tantric sex lead to prolonged orgasmic experiences?

Yes, tantric sex can lead to prolonged orgasmic experiences. Tantra is an ancient practice that combines elements of spirituality, meditation, and sexual techniques to promote a deep connection between partners and increased awareness of one's body and pleasure. The goal of tantric sex is not only to achieve orgasm but also to explore and amplify pleasure through specific techniques and intense emotional and physical connection.

Elements of Tantric Sex

1. **Mindful Breathing:** Breathing deeply and in sync with your partner helps relax the body, increase sexual energy, and create a sense of union.

2. **Slow and Intentional Movements:** Slow, deliberate movements allow partners to experience each sensation more intensely, extending pleasure and leading to prolonged arousal.

3. **Eye Contact:** Maintaining eye contact strengthens the emotional connection between partners, amplifying feelings of pleasure and union.

4. **Meditation and Mindfulness:** Incorporating meditation and mindfulness practices into tantric sex helps

focus on the present moment, reducing distractions, and increasing awareness of bodily sensations.

5.   **Body Exploration:** Exploring the partner's body with attention and care, touching and massaging slowly, can increase pleasure and prolong arousal.

Prolonged Orgasmic Experiences

1.   **Orgasm Control:** Tantra teaches orgasm control through breathing and muscle contraction, helping delay orgasm and prolong pleasure.

2.   **Multiple Orgasms:** Tantra can facilitate multiple orgasms by combining techniques that maintain arousal without immediately reaching climax.

3.   **Full-Body Orgasm:** Tantra aims to spread orgasmic energy throughout the body rather than concentrating it only in the genitals, leading to a more intense and prolonged sensation of pleasure.

4.   **States of Ecstasy:** The practice of tantra can lead to deep states of ecstasy, where pleasure extends beyond the physical and involves the mind and spirit, lasting longer than traditional orgasms.

How to Practice Tantric Sex

1.   **Preparation:** Create a quiet, relaxing environment free from distractions. Soft lighting, scented candles, and relaxing music can help set the right mood.

2.   **Open Communication:** Talk with your partner about your expectations and desires. Open communication is essential for successful tantric practice.

3.   **Breathing Techniques:** Start with breathing exercises to sync your breath with your partner. This helps establish a deep connection and prepare the body and mind.

4.   **Slow and Mindful Exploration:** Take time to explore your partner's body with slow touches and caresses. Focus on each sensation and remain present in the moment.

5.   **Building Arousal:** Alternate between moments of intense stimulation and calm. This helps build arousal without immediately reaching orgasm.

Can sex be a spiritual experience?

Yes, sex can certainly be a spiritual experience for many people. The connection between sexuality and spirituality has been a theme across various cultures, religions, and philosophies for millennia. Here are some ways in which sex can be experienced as a spiritual experience:

1. Deep Connection with the Partner

Emotional and Physical Intimacy:

Sex can create a profound sense of intimacy between partners. This intimacy can go beyond mere physical pleasure, promoting a sense of unity and connection that can be experienced as spiritual.

Vulnerability and Trust:

Being physically and emotionally vulnerable with a partner can foster a spiritual connection. The trust and openness developed in this context can lead to a feeling of unity and transcendence. **2. Spiritual Practices and Traditions**

Tantra:

Tantra is a spiritual practice that views sexuality as a means to achieve enlightenment and transcendence. Through breathing techniques, movement, and meditation, Tantra seeks to harmonize the body, mind, and spirit, using sexual energy as a tool for personal and spiritual growth.

Taoism:

Taoism has a similar view, considering sex as a way to balance the yin and yang energies in the body. Taoist practices of "sexual alchemy" aim to improve health, longevity, and spirituality through conscious management of sexual energy.

3.Individual Experiences of Transcendence

Ecstasy and Transformation:

For some people, sex can induce states of ecstasy comparable to spiritual experiences. These states can include a sense of merging with the partner, loss of self, and connection to something greater.

Awareness and Presence:

Being fully present during the sexual act, paying attention to every sensation and emotion, can transform the experience into a moment of awareness and meditation. This presence can elevate the sexual act to a spiritual level.

4.Sexual Energy as Life Force

Kundalini:

In yoga tradition, sexual energy is often identified with Kundalini energy, a life force said to reside at the base of the spine. When awakened through sexual and spiritual practices, this energy can ascend along the spine, leading to elevated states of consciousness.

Creativity and Expression:

Sexual energy is also seen as a creative force. Its expression is not only physical but also emotional and spiritual, and it can manifest in various forms of creativity and self-expression.

5.Rites and Ceremonies

Union Rituals:

In many cultures, sex is incorporated into rites of passage and ceremonies celebrating the union of two individuals. These rituals can have profound spiritual significance, symbolizing the union of souls as well as bodies.

6.Overcoming Dualities

Unity and Non-Duality:

Sex can be seen as a means to overcome the duality between self and other, body and spirit, earthly and divine. In this context, the sexual act can become an experience of unity and non-duality, reflecting the interconnected nature of all existence.

Sex can be much more than a physical act; it can become an experience of deep connection, awareness, and transcendence. Through specific practices like Tantra or simply through an attitude of presence and openness, the sexual act can transform into a moment of spirituality and personal growth. The key lies in the conscious approach and mutual respect between partners, recognizing the sacred potential of sexual energy.

Conclusion

This book has explored a wide range of topics related to human sexuality, offering information, advice, and reflections for living a more conscious and fulfilling intimate life. From techniques to improve sexual experiences to exploring fantasies and desires, from managing difficulties like decreased desire or anorgasmia, to the importance of communication and mutual respect, this book has aimed to provide tools for a freer, more aware, and joyful sexuality.

The author hopes that the discussion of these topics, direct and without taboos as it may be, has not offended the sensibilities of any reader. The purpose of this book is solely informative and educational, with the goal of providing a complete and conscious view of human sexuality.

We remind you that every individual is unique, and there is no "magic formula" applicable to all. The key to a fulfilling sexual life lies in listening to oneself, one's body, and one's desires, in open and honest communication with the partner, and in the willingness to explore, experiment, and grow together.

If this book has sparked new curiosities, doubts, or the need for personalized support, do not hesitate to contact qualified professionals such as sexologists or couple therapists, who can accompany you on a journey of discovery and personal growth.

In this book, we have seen that sex is not just a physical act or a means of pleasure; it can be a gateway to deeper and more meaningful experiences. Through sex, one can achieve a unique connection not only with the partner but also with a higher dimension of being that transcends the everyday. This spiritual connection is not reserved only for esoteric practices like Tantra or Taoism but can be experienced by anyone with awareness and openness.

The spirituality in sex can manifest in various ways: in the deep intimacy and emotional union with the partner, in the awareness of the present moment that transforms every touch and sensation into a meditative act, and in the creative energy that is released through the sexual act, akin to a life force that nourishes body and spirit.

Being vulnerable and authentic during the sexual act, allowing ourselves to be completely present and open, can lead to experiences of transcendence. These moments can become true rites of passage that strengthen the bond between partners and with the divine, awakening a sense of unity and non-duality.

In a world that often reduces sex to a mere physical act or performance, rediscovering its spiritual dimension can offer us a new perspective, enriching our lives and those of our partners. The awareness that sex can be sacred and transformative invites us to live this experience with respect, gratitude, and love.

Sex is much more than what appears on the surface. It is a complex journey that can lead us to new depths of connection and understanding. Whether it is exploring new techniques, openly communicating with the partner, or embracing the spirituality of sex, each step we take towards greater awareness and intimacy brings us closer to living a fuller and more integrated life.

With this awareness, we can celebrate sex not only as an act of pleasure but as a sacred dance that nourishes the body, mind, and soul.